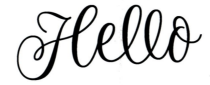

this is for you,
your loved ones,
your students

B. Smith 7 months ago

Thank you thank you thank you. I've wanted to do this for 10 years and I didn't understand the books I read and have to travel to find a practitioner.

Kate Major 1 year ago

Such an excellent explanation. The fact you can explain it so clearly gives me the confidence that you know your material [..] This is very socially conscious of you to make excellent teaching available to those who want to practice but can not travel to classes or in some cases, afford full fees.

Linda Clark 7 months ago

I have heard about this method a long time ago but thanks to Youtube and Alfons I get to get lessons in it. So exciting for me.

Phil Gardner 1 year ago

Hi Alfons, I understand what you said about this not being a medical institution and that you aren't a doctor. And I don't expect 'the' answers to all questions, but I think people turn to people like you for answers because they have already been to physiotherapists, doctors, and various 'experts' and didn't receive the help they needed. That doesn't mean you are responsible for the health of others, but I just wanted to give you this feedback, because I would trust your advice more than many others, simply because you are helping people to learn for themselves (which helps everyone), and not just giving information for people to consume (which might be right for some, but not for others).

FB 5 months ago

This is all new to me...Somatic...but I'm already hooked on Alfons. Excellent explanations and demonstrations. How do I subscribe?

All testimonial citations in the preface are from publicly visible comments in the public comment section of my YouTube video „GETTING BETTER DAY BY DAY: INTRODUCTION", https://goo.gl/aDixwc, (December 10, 2017). I try to attribute as correctly as feasible, according to the official APA guidelines.

„Feldenkrais With Alfons – Getting Better Day By Day – The Workbook" written by Alfons Grabher

Copyright © Alfons Grabher,
All rights reserved.
1st edition December 2017

www.myfeldenkraisbook.com
info@feldenkraiswerkstatt.at
6900 Bregenz, Austria, Europe

Alfons Grabher is a certified FELDENKRAIS® Practitioner, born in 1974 in Vienna, Austria, Europe. He also is a graduate Engineer (University of Applied Sciences, Vienna), specialized in Biomedical Engineering. Prior to becoming a FELDENKRAIS® Practitioner he has worked for over a decade as Software Engineer and Consultant.

In Austria the Feldenkrais® Verband Österreich (FVÖ) is responsible for the trademarks for „FELDENKRAIS®" and „Der/die FVÖ zertifizierte/r Feldenkrais-LehrererIn®".
„Feldenkrais Method®" is a registered trademark in the U.K. of the Feldenkrais Guild UK Ltd., Reg No. 1563759.
Feldenkrais®, Feldenkrais Method®, Functional Integration®, Awareness Through Movement®, and Guild Certified Feldenkrais Practitioner^{cm} are service marks in the United States of the FELDENKRAIS GUILD® of North America.

The information in this book is given in good faith and strictly for reference only and is neither intended to diagnose any physical or mental condition nor to serve as a substitute for medical advice or professional health care. Please remember that no practice can be adequately learned from written descriptions. Talk to your doctor before starting any new exercise regime.

Mention of specific companies, organizations or authorities in this book does not imply endorsement by the author, nor does mention of specific companies, organizations or authorities imply that they endorse this book or its author.

Internet addresses in this book were accurate at the time it was uploaded to the printing service.
Note from Alfons: not all notes in this workbook correspond 1:1 to what I've said in the videos. Furthermore there's no guarantee for the availability of my videos on YouTube. However I try my best to keep the videos online and easy to find.

Limon Font Family by Typesenses (Sabrina Mariela Lopez)
Debby Free Font by Artimasa and Free Design Resources
Inhabitants Npc Sloth by glitch

Printed by CreateSpace, An Amazon.com Company
ISBN-13: 978-1981641932
ISBN-10: 1981641939

FOREWORD

My dear reader, student, client, friend, follower, subscriber. I'll try to keep the foreword short and sweet:

1. The human nervous system is the most complex, most mysterious, and most astonishing object in the known universe. And you're using it right now. How amazing is that?

2. I simply love the fact that you're interested in the FELDENKRAIS® Method of Somatic Education, and my movement lessons. I belief that the FELDENKRAIS® Method – which was invented by and named after the exceptionally brilliant Dr. Moshé Feldenkrais (1904-1984) – is one of the great achievements of humanity. And a fairly recent achievement that is. It seems like it took all the millions and thousands of years of evolution to enable us humans to create and to appreciate this method. It's definitely a stepping stone to a deeper understanding of ourselves, the world, and everyone else. I believe that we will see much more of it in the future.

3. I originally created the „Getting Better Day By Day" lessons as a video course, available for free on YouTube. This online video course is intended for beginners as well as movement professionals, and accessible to anyone with an Internet connection. Only later I created this workbook... in fact, this 118 pages workbook was more than a year in the making. My hope is that this workbook will enable you to get a quick overview over the lessons, a better understanding of the connections between lessons, and that you'll be able to identify the strategies used in the lessons easier. And that you have something to show to your people when you're trying to explain what you're doing (in case they're worrying why you're rolling on the floor in seemingly random, slow motion movements). You can use this workbook to deepen your own practice and understanding, or use it as teaching material to get others to roll on the floor and feel hilariously peaceful ... piece ... in one piece ... complete. Yes. We can be.

4. In this workbook I tried to use the same light, colloquial, yet sincere and authentic spirit I show in my videos. I hope this does not throw you off. It still is a very serious method – and a thoroughly designed, serious workbook. My ability to create this workbook is thanks to my professional education, my 10+ years teaching experience, and the many students I have had the opportunity to work with in person. This course can be and has been life changing. It's just that the good, life changing stuff don't need to be that serious. Even though it is.

5. Did I already mention that you're amazing?

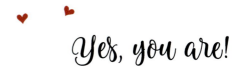

I wish you a great time on the floor, and
„See you in the next video!"
Alfons

TABLE OF CONTENTS

Skyler Shelton 11 months ago

Thank you for the wonderful lesson! I totally deserve feeling great today :)

1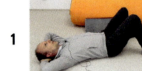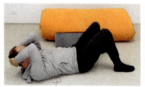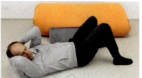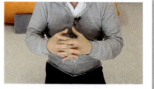

LIFTING YOUR HEAD IN SUPINE POSITION Page 10

2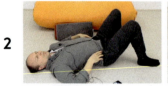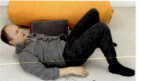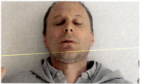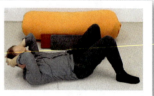

YOUR EYES AND YOUR PELVIS HELP LIFTING YOUR HEAD Page 20

3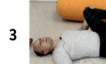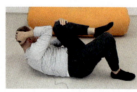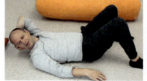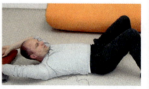

ELBOWS TOWARDS KNEES Page 32

4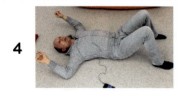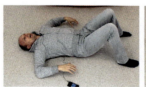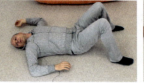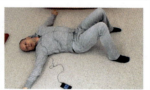

GETTING TO KNOW YOUR SHOULDER GIRDLE AND ITS CONNECTIONS TO THE WHOLE BODY Page 44

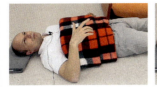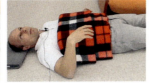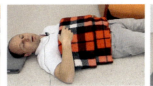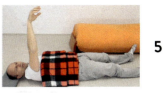

FLOATING AND LENGTHENING, STARTING WITH YOUR DOMINANT HAND — 5 — Page 56

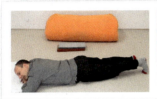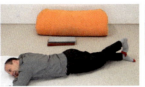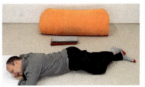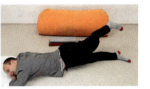

LIFTING YOUR LEGS IN PRONE POSITION — 6 — Page 68

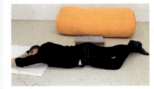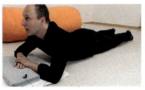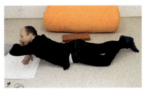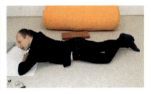

LIFTING YOUR HEAD IN PRONE POSITION — 7 — Page 80

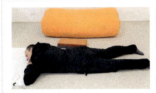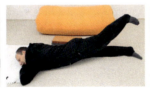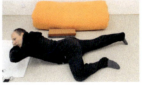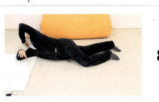

ROLLING OVER EASILY, USING EVERYTHING YOU'VE GOT — 8 — Page 92

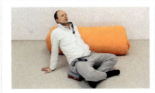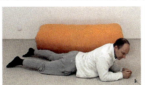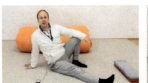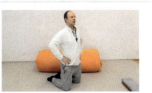

FLEXION & EXTENSION IN 16 DIFFERENT POSITIONS — 9 — Page 108

Penthesilea — 1 month ago

I am fortunate enough to have the time to do your videos several times per day so I have an opportunity to explore the movements the way you suggest. I have been doing this one many times. Today, I chose to try to lift my head without using any unnecessary muscles or other bodily aids (in line with some of your other suggestions). I could not lift my head at all. I thought about the things I learned from you and decided to try to initiate the movement with my eyes looking toward the ceiling. Lo and behold, my head moved up using the barest whisper of muscles in my neck, chest, upper back and shoulders. I used this technique throughout the lesson. I am so pleased with the results that I wanted to tell you about it. This is a very excited journey. Many thanks again, Alfons.

Luisa Moreno — 1 year ago

thank you, the introduction made me laugh like crazy..... that is a fix in itself

Ntathu Allen — 1 year ago

I feel very regal and graceful. Makes a big difference when you said to be aware of the space between the floor and the head. Thank you. Maybe you could "market this sequence" as how to improve your posture" or tips to ease neck ache from slouching all day at computer? because I definitely feel more open and square across the chest and my posture and head neck and back alignment improved. And yes...I do feel better for doing this sequence. Thanks for all you do.

Fiama — 11 months ago

Your unperfectness and humor make me happy. Thank you for your natural authenticity

Sarah Gray — 10 months ago

I love these videos. They are so lighthearted and relaxing and they make a difference and make me smile. Thanks Alfons!

Anita Acevedo — 3 months ago

Thank you, Alfons, for being so generous with us via youtube. I practice your videos more regularly now and I notice feeling like my movements are more supple and fluid - your transparency is uniquely you and makes the lessons almost like being with you in person!

Newman Lanier — 1 year ago

Thank you. Thank you. Thank you! I've been using your videos all summer with much benefit. looking forward to a winter of exploring movement and awareness with you and everyone here. Serveus aus California, Newman

cofycup — 9 months ago

I certainly felt that my neck could move through its rotations much more smoothly, as if the movement was using muscles it hadn't been using before, and not using others that it had been. It was quite a pleasurable sensation of freedom. Thank you.

Kevin Curtin — 1 year ago

Great new sequence, Alfons. You are taking us back to first principals to integrate the whole body's movement train to lift the head. You don't really want or need a snappy title here, because you are aiming for integration from the sole of the feet on up to the head. Just the deviation move from midline, and the shifts with the elbow gave me a profound new sense of the head and neck, chest, shoulders, ribs and vertebrae. You have got it all going on, and I look forward to the next lesson in the train. Oh, and my head does float much better over the top of the spine. Best, Kevin in Maine

Catherine T — 2 months ago

thanks Alfons. Just found and started going through your videos. They make me smile and physically the few i have done feel good!

Liz Torres — 9 months ago

I found your channel "by chance" and I can not express well enough how much I was needing this. Thank you for your lessons and I just finished this one and I felt as if I was actually having a conversation with you, like being in the same room practicing, I laughed and enjoyed it so much!! Liz

All testimonial citations in this chapter are from publicly visible comments in the public comment section of my YouTube video „FIX FORWARD NECK POSTURE WITH THIS UNUSUAL APPROACH?", https://goo.gl/XC4QHp, (December 3, 2017). I try to attribute as correctly as feasible, according to the official APA guidelines.

LESSON 1

Lifting your head in supine position

Haley Myles — 1 month ago

Thank you, Alfons, for this wonderful lesson! I am looking forward to going through your "Getting Better Day by Day" sequence. I am new to the Feldenkrais method and I am amazed what a difference I feel after half an hour of slight movements.

Sue Hall — 8 months ago

I just started doing your program and am committing to follow a lesson every day and leaving a comment daily on how my progress is going. I have Lyme Disease and a lot of chronic pain and am unable to go to classes so I am happy to have found your program. I will be ordering your book which I found on Amazon. Thanks for doing all these wonderful videos.

Testimonials show how your virtual classmates are doing

YouTube videos always need to have a catchy title

Thumbnail images give you quick, visual cues

Bold, uppercase titles let you know what to do in a glance

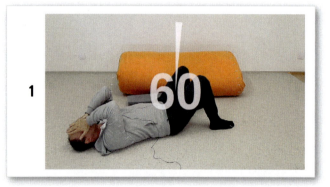

ARRIVE ON THE FLOOR

Get on the floor and give yourself a minute or two to really arrive on the floor. What is the meaning of this? What needs to be happening? How long does it take to truly „arrive" on the floor, and why is that? Why is a change of position not always instantaneously accompanied by change of muscle tonus?

Images have a sequential number to make it easier for you to keep track of the movements

A brief description reminds you of basic details and questions to ask

PLEASE WORK THROUGH THE *VIDEO FIRST* **TO BENEFIT FULLY FROM THIS** *Workbook*

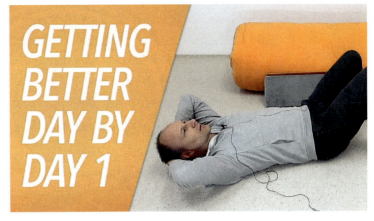

YOUTUBE VIDEO TITLE:
FIX FORWARD NECK POSTURE WITH THIS UNUSUAL APPROACH?

In this lesson you will explore how to lift your head in great detail, in supine position (which means to rest on your back). This is a somewhat similar movement to lowering your head in an upright position. However, when you're in a supine position there are a number of peculiarities:

GRAVITY

In supine position you are in a different orientation towards gravity than when you're in an upright position. This in itself is quite astounding. We humans are not build from the ground up, but grown from inside out (if that makes any sense). Our body mechanics are not the same as the mechanics for man made objects. Rather, we would have to speak in terms of biotensegrity and soft matter physics. It's not possible to turn a building, a car or even a bicycle on it's side or upside down, and expect it to continue to function properly. This is different for us humans: simple changes in posture don't break us apart. Even better, every new posture comes with new possibilities. For example: when we lie down on the floor we don't break, but we can roll. Or just rest the head. Or examine how to lift the head in great detail. When lying down we don't have to deal with gravity and balance in the same way as in, for example, standing, sitting, squatting, kneeling or even side lying. We can't fall, because we're already lying down. Therefore, we're freed up to focus on the finer details of movement. Moving mindfully and slowly through meaningful, well thought out movement sequences, and with frequent rests, will make for a somatic experience.

POSSIBILITIES

Each new position brings a new set of possibilites. For example, in lying supine the chest can't expand backwards very well. Breathing against the floor is harder than breathing into the empty space in front of you and to your sides. Contrariwise, in lying prone (belly on the floor) it's easier to expand the chest backwards, since in that situation there's no floor to constrict your breathing in your back. When you're lying on your left side, you can't easily bend your head to the left (because there's the floor), but when you lift your head in a side bending movement to the right, you will be able to feel how you lean against the floor with your left side. Left, right, up, down, sounds complicated? Let's better get to the lessons soon, everything will become clear as you line up your movements, thinking, feeling and sensing at the same time.

SMOOTHNESS

There's many things to learn and to take home from this first lesson. It's impossible to list all of them, alas, impossible to even think of them all. In FELDENKRAIS® lessons you will always get more than you expect. Basically it's up to you to find what is interesting for you at the moment.

Having that said, one of the things you will learn might well be: How lifting your head is connected with the movements of your neck, chest and actually your entire spine, right down to your pelvis and feet.

This will make you (1) more aware of yourself, and (2) make your spine movements smoother and (3) better distributed throughout your whole self. In this sense it's a blessing for neck related issues, like limited range of movement, neck pain due to poor movement mechanics, being stuck in a forward head posture, issues related to high muscle tension and much more.

Let us begin, shall we?

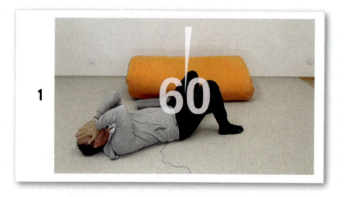

ARRIVE ON THE FLOOR
Get on the floor and give yourself a minute or two to really arrive on the floor. What is the meaning of this? What needs to be happening? How long does it take to truly „arrive" on the floor, and why is that? Why is a change of position not always instantaneously accompanied by change of muscle tonus?

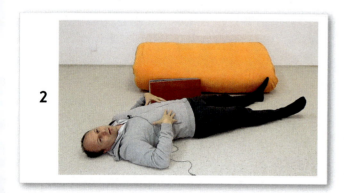

SCAN FOR POINTS OF CONTACT
Legs extended. Do a scan: where do you touch the floor? Where do you not touch the floor? Check for example: your heels, calves, behind your knees, the small of your back. How strong of a pressure against the floor do you feel at these various locations? How big of a contact area is there? How do similar parts compare to each other, for example, your right shoulder blade compared to your left shoulder blade?

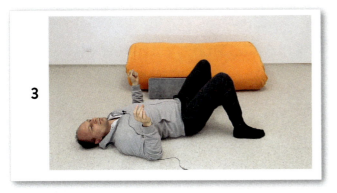

SCAN AGAIN, WITH FEET STANDING

Stand your feet. Repeat the previous observations. What's different now in this position with your knees bent and your feet standing? Where is more or less pressure, more or less effort? (e. g. your legs, small of your back, jaw, breathing, back of your chest, etc.)

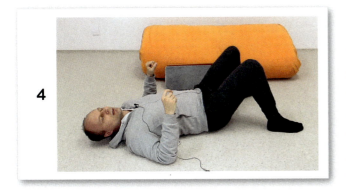

LIFT YOUR HEAD

Lift your head a bit to see how it is – this is the so called „reference movement". We will try this movement again later to see if and how it has changed. Be sure that your feet are standing. If you don't know or can't feel why they should be standing, try this lesson with your legs long and try to discover the difference it makes.

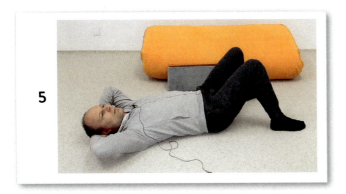

LIFT YOUR HEAD WITH THE HELP OF YOUR HANDS & ARMS

Interlace your hands and rest your head (not your neck) in your interlaced hands. Then lift your head with the help of your neck and upper body. Alternately, let your head be lifted by your hands and arms. Feel the difference. Lift it just a bit, not to the maximum.

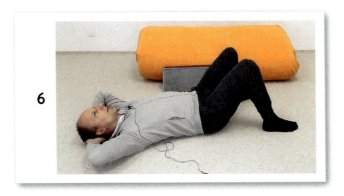

LIFT YOUR HEAD WITH YOUR ELBOWS POINTING OUTWARDS

Next time you lift your head make sure your elbows are pointing outwards. Try again, slowly.

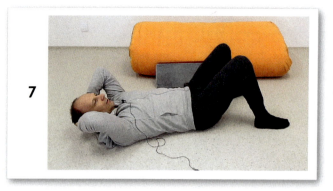

LIFT YOUR HEAD WITH ELBOWS TILTED HALFWAY UP

Lift your head with your elbows in a 45° angle from the floor. How is that different?

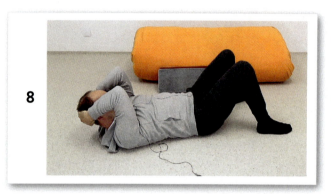

LIFT YOUR HEAD WITH ELBOWS POINTING TOWARDS THE CEILING

From now on make this your default way to hold your elbows when lifting your head (why?).

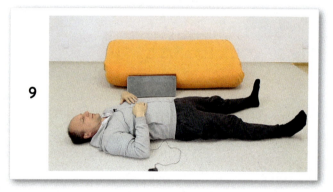

REST AND OBSERVE

Can you feel that your shoulder area changed in the way it rests on the floor? How lightly or heavily is your head resting on the floor now? Notice anything else?

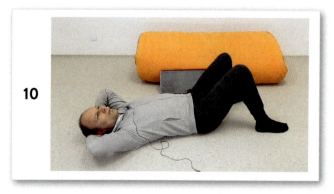

OBSERVE YOUR BREATHING

Interlace your hands again and rest your head (not your neck) in your interlaced hands. Observe your breathing. When do you breath in? Is there a pause after the in-breath? When do you breath out? Is there a pause after the out-breath? Do not change your breathing, merely observe.

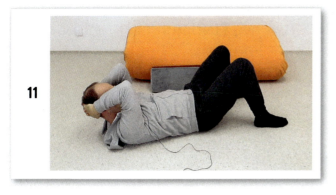

SYNC YOUR BREATHING AND LIFTING OF YOUR HEAD

Wait for it. Just like the surfer waits for the wave. Lift your head on an out-breath. Lift your head on an in-breath. Lift your head while holding your breath. Always compare.

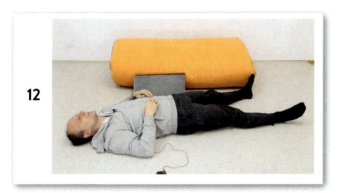

REST, OBSERVE

Have a short rest. During the rest feel the reverberation of the previous movements. This kind of rest is similar to the silence after a piece of music or a poem. It's very subtle, but it's there. Ask yourself: where was effort in this movement? How could it be done easier? How do I feel?

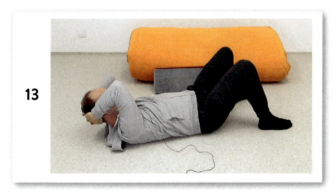

TARGET YOUR LEFT KNEE WITH YOUR RIGHT ELBOW

Lift your head again but add a little bit of a twist, so that you target your left knee with your right elbow while lifting your head. Just a bit. Don't go crazy. Don't do funny contortions or even worse: twisting sit ups. Lift your head just a bit, and discover how and where you are twisting.

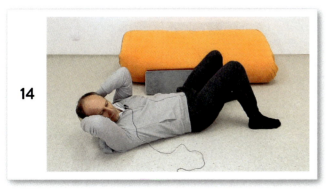

TARGET YOUR RIGHT KNEE WITH YOUR LEFT ELBOW

Keep the extend of the rotation small, somewhere between one and thirty degrees (or so). Stay in your comfort zone. Make small, enjoyable movements. Take plenty of rests in between. Think, move, feel, sense. Rest.

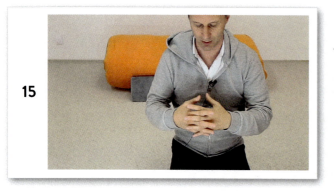

INTERLACING FINGERS TECHNIQUE
What's your preferred way to interlace your fingers? Right or left thumb on top? Which way feels more familiar?

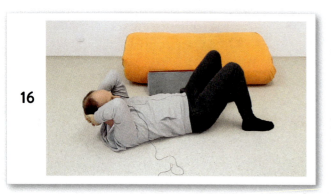

LIFT YOUR HEAD
WITH YOUR FINGERS INTERLACED
IN THE LESS FAMILIAR WAY
How does this feel different? Does it change how you lift your head? Does it change how much or what you sense?

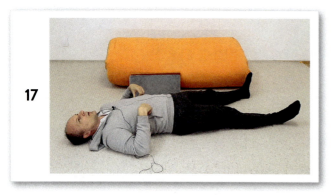

REST, OBSERVE

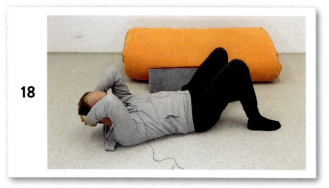

PEEL YOUR HEAD FROM THE FLOOR
Lift your head again but this time, instead of paying attention to your head, pay attention to the space between yourself (head, cervical spine, shoulders) and the floor. This space is getting bigger the further you're into lifting your head. Some people find the image of peeling a sticker off from a window helpful. Every half inch is a success!

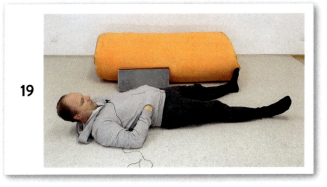

LIFT HEAD – REFERENCE MOVEMENT
Lift your head again and observe how it is now compared to the beginning [4].

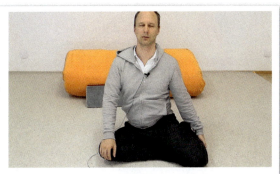

SIT UP
Come to sit. Move your head around a bit. Feel how you carry your head.

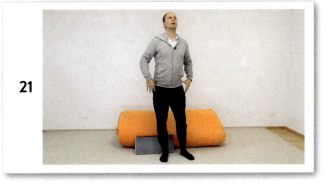

STAND UP
Come to stand, observe how you carry your head. Feel your shoulders, pelvis, your feet, how your weight is distributed over your left foot, your right foot, how you balance yourself on top of your feet. Move your head around a bit, move with your head. Feel how it is.

John Moseley 1 month ago

Wow. Dramatic difference between how I lifted my head at the start and end. Quite difficult at the start, very easy at the end. Also, lots of tension in the back of the neck and shoulders gone. Brilliant. Thank you.

pablo fabregas 3 months ago

Just finished your lesson, Alfonse. When you said, "Wonderful" in the end of the lesson that was exactly what I was thinking. Really feel like my head is floating on top of my spine. I'm suddenly so aware of the distance between my head and my shoulders and everything. My neck feels so long! Giraffe-like.

Gustavo Oliva 5 months ago

wonderful feeling !! enjoyed this first lesos!! thanks Alfons!

kira mango 10 months ago

Thank you for saying that it's an achievement to lie down without pain and that it can take awhile to get there

KS 7 months ago

Great one. I enjoyed every second... love the opportunity for proprioceptive feedback. Look forward to more!

Theo Herren 3 weeks ago

I was amazed, standing up and walking around after the exercise to what an extent my whole posture had changed, how tall and upright I was standing, walking. An amazing experience at age 79! Thanks a lot Alfons for putting your whole heart and soul into doing and teaching and Feldenkrais exercises.

Henry Thomas 10 months ago

I am laughing a bit, because last lesson and in this lesson too I had so much tension in my neck and spine under my shoulders when trying to lift my head. But at the end of this lesson, I tried to lift my head again as you said, and nearly no tension at all! Incredible! I am going to continue through the 10 days. I am so happy to have learned about Feldenkrais through your channel here. :-)

smrkit 1 year ago

Very interesting. Feel refreshed and I don't know why. Intriguing

Linda Cantor 4 months ago

Ah-h-h. I love the phrase carry your head. It reminds me of "think of a sky hook holding you by the head". These lessons are. Making me aware of my movements throughout the day, and I feel more integrated with my body. Thank you. Also, at the beginning I couldn't even lift my head off the floor. Amazing results from simplicity.

Olga Shmidov 1 year ago

Thank you again for excellent lesson!!!! I felt a waves of energy in my body just from moving eyes up... I do and work with energy , but my big surprise was that they started from neck..... (usually from lower part of body) is there any explanations for that? Thank you.

MXB67 4 months ago

In this exercise I felt my rib joints connecting with the spine gained in the range of motion. They kept crackling all the way through excercise. Completely different result against expectation of chest muscles release. It also gave me good spine massage.

Skyler Shelton 11 months ago

Thank you for the wonderful lesson! I totally deserve feeling great today :)

Penthesilea 2 months ago

I just wanted to lift my head but my entire T Spine came up with it! In the past I had to contort all my muscles just to get my shoulder blades off the ground and now they fly up. Thanks!

Haley Myles 1 month ago

I feel reinvigorated and relaxed. Thanks so much. Also - nice touch using the Goldberg Variations. ;)

allonespiriti 1 month ago

I have been chronically ill for 7 years in bed a lot. I can do these and not rush and make smaller or less movements. Its great!

The connection with eyes and head movements is very interesting ! I found it was much easier to roll the eyeballs if I stop trying to see and focused on the sensation of eye movement.

Sue Hall 8 months ago

Thank you again for these amazing videos. I love your style and humour as well as your professionalism in the way you describe what to do. I am so looking forward to doing all your lessons.

Phil Gardner 1 year ago

Nice lesson. I wonder if one way to help smooth the eye movements is to move the head while fixing the eyes on a distant point. Then I found the movement to be very smooth. The body floating sensation at the end is a very nice way to see the effects of the lesson. Thank you.

All testimonial citations in this chapter are from publicly visible comments in the public comment section of my YouTube video „A CHEST OPENER WITHOUT STRETCHING (EYE MOVEMENTS)", https://goo.gl/hUxHkP, (December 3, 2017). I try to attribute as correctly as feasible, according to the official APA guidelines.

LESSON 2

Your eyes & your pelvis help lifting your head

Rest until you feel like playing, then play until you feel like resting.

MARTHA BECK

PLEASE WORK THROUGH THE
VIDEO FIRST
TO BENEFIT FULLY FROM THIS
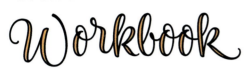

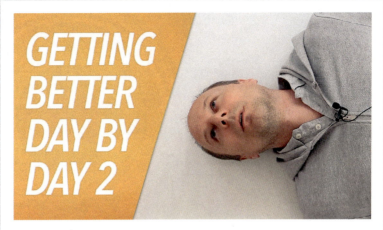

YOUTUBE VIDEO TITLE:
A CHEST OPENER WITHOUT STRETCHING (EYE MOVEMENTS)

In this lesson you'll briefly review the previous lesson and then start adding a pelvic tilt to the repertoire (or in modern speak: movement vocabulary). Then specific eye movements are introduced, and finally everything is put together. backwards and forwards, and how this goes together with lifting the head in supine position. And best of all, how all of this is connected to eye movements. You will re-discover meaningful ways of how to train your eyes. Exciting!

ROLLING

Pelvic movements and how they relate, affect and distribute to other areas of the body are a big topic in FELDENKRAIS® lessons. The encapsulating theme is called „pelvic clock". If you're an experienced FELDENKRAIS® student you surely already came across one or the other pelvic clock lesson. In this lesson we'll look at the anterior and posterior pelvic tilt, which means to roll your pelvis

QUALITY

The eyes are not just for seeing. Amongst other things, they direct movement. Every muscle and bone in your body, however big or small, everything, is following the lead of your eyes (unless you're blind). The way you use your eyes does support, disturb, affect, direct the general quality of all your movements. But don't just take my word for it, try it for *yourself* ♡

ARRIVE ON THE FLOOR
Get on the floor and give yourself a minute or two to relax to the floor more completely.

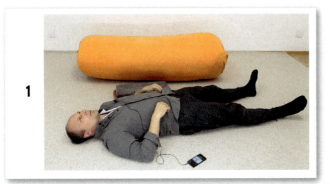

1

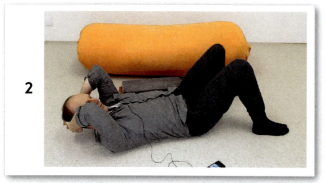

RECAP THE PREVIOUS LESSON
Move through a couple of things you remember from the previous lesson. Focus not only on the movements themselves, but also try to recall what you have learned, experienced, felt, sensed, noticed, what you were thinking during the lesson. Movements are merely movements. However, your somatic experiencing – and all that comes with it – is unique, and should be celebrated as such.

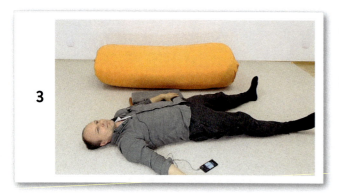

TAKE A SHORT REST
Scan, feel, breath, feel the aftereffects of what you just did, sensed, thought, experienced.

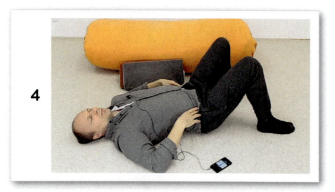

ROLL YOUR PELVIS FORWARDS
Roll your pelvis forwards, towards your tailbone. This direction is called „anterior". Do this many times. It's not like you do roll into a back bridge pose, it's just the pelvis rolling a tiny little bit.

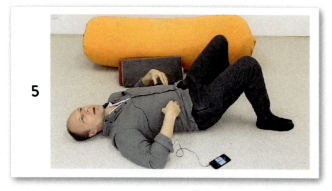

ROLL YOUR PELVIS BACKWARDS
Roll your pelvis backwards, towards your chest. This is called „posterior". Then let the pelvis fall back into neutral.

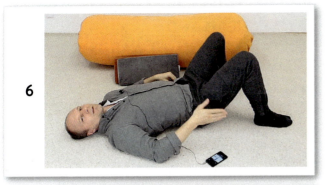

COMBINE: ROLL PELVIS FORWARDS THEN BACKWARDS

Combine the two previous movements into one fluid motion.

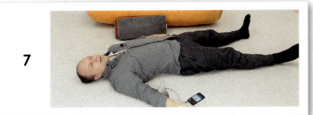

REST

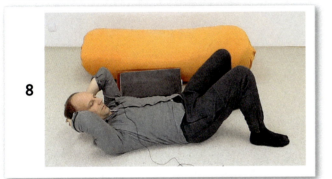

LIFT YOUR HEAD AGAIN

Lift any way you like, explore, play for a bit, compare to how it was before, and how having become more aware of your pelvis enhances your experience of lifting the head.

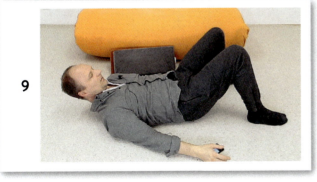

LIFT YOUR HEAD WITHOUT THE HELP OF YOUR ARMS

Rest your arms on the floor and compare how the lifting works now. Remember, we experimented with this difference in the previous lesson already. Now we are comparing how this difference developed through time and experience.

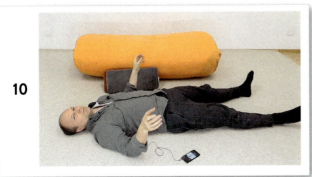

TAKE ANOTHER REST

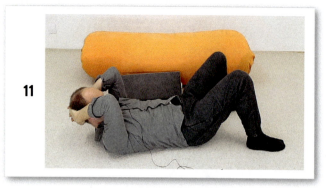

LIFT YOUR HEAD AND ROLL YOUR PELVIS BACKWARDS

Combine those two motions as they naturally come together, or combine them intentionally, on purpose. Play with movement initiation, what moves first? Explore as well as direct.

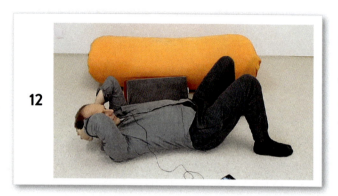

LIFT YOUR HEAD AND ROLL YOUR PELVIS FORWARDS

Try this unusual combination, which might feel rather crazy at first try. Try to get comfortable with it, then try to get better at it.

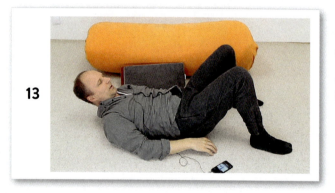

LIFT YOUR HEAD AGAIN

With your arms resting on the floor lift your head again any way you like, play for a bit, compare to before.

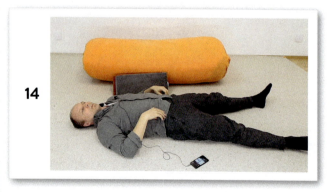

TAKE A SHORT REST

Think about the previous movements and how they echo into your resting position.

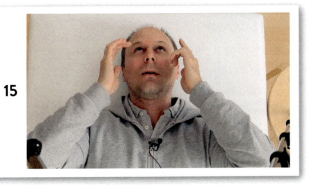

EYES UPWARDS

Lie on your back in a supine position, have your feet standing (with your knees pointing towards the ceiling). Roll your eyes upwards, and let go again (let them drop back to neutral). Try this many times. Try to make it simpler, more fluent.

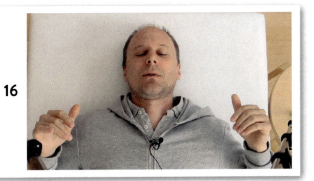

EYES DOWNWARDS

This time roll your eyeballs downwards. Or think of looking downwards to your feet. Roll your eyeballs gradually. Don't make big jumps. Notice where you have „blind spots".

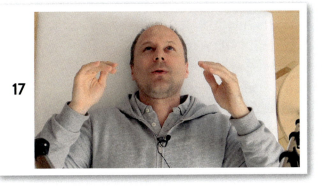

COMBINE: ROLL EYES UPWARDS AND THEN DOWNWARDS

Now combine both directions. Always let your eyes fall back to neutral. Where is neutral? In which position are your eyes neither rolled up nor rolled down?

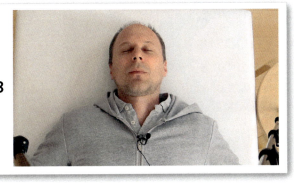

REST

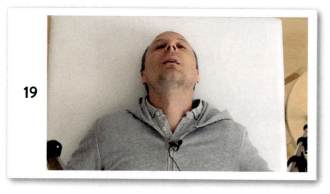

NOD HEAD UP

Instead of rolling your eyes up, roll your head up, in a movement like „nodding", raise your head slightly and briefly. Maybe think of your nose going up, or the back of your head going down. Always come back to your „home" position, don't nod down just yet.

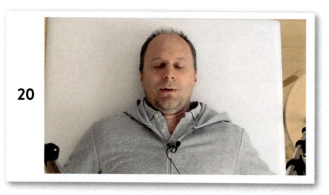

NOD HEAD DOWN

Try to make smooth, not jerky movements. Notice where you direct your awareness to, how you do think about this movement.

1. Think   2. Move   3. Sense   4. Feel

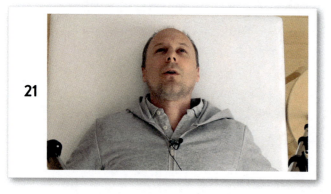

COMBINE: NOD HEAD UP AND THEN DOWN

Combine these two directions. There are many things to notice. Where is the neutral position? Try up first, then down. Then try down first, then up. Are there differences? What kind of differences?

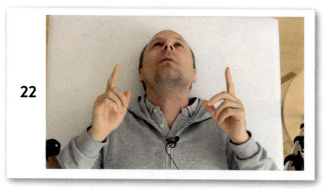

COMBINE: ROLL EYES UPWARDS AND NOD HEAD UP

Combine the previous movements: roll your eyeballs upwards and at the same time, with the same speed, and to the same extend nod your head upwards

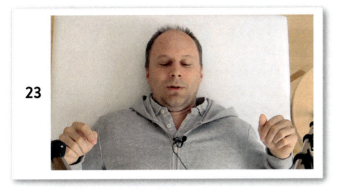

COMBINE: ROLL EYES DOWNWARDS AND NOD HEAD DOWN

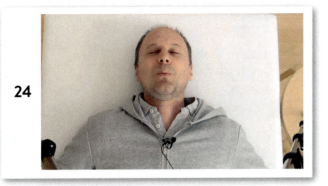

REST

Such eye movements can be very strenuous. Never underestimate that strain that you put on your eyes. Your eyes are your precious, treat them well and give them a good rest after a set of unusual movements These movements have the power to facilitate a lot of change. Take rests as you need them. Cover your eyes with the palms of your hands if you like to.

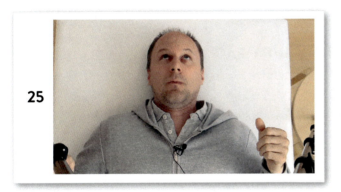

EYES AND HEAD IN OPPOSITE DIRECTIONS

In FELDENKRAIS® we call this technique „differentiation". We distinguish, separate, set apart. This means that we not only make a conscious attempt at thinking, moving, sensing and feeling, but we use actual „differentiating movements" to help us become aware of what is going on. In other words we use this kind of differentiation to uncover the elusive, and create inroads to ourselves that would otherwise be very hard to establish and almost impossible to improve upon. This is one of the big secrets of this method, you struck gold! We're not going too deep here, just a brief differentiation. Roll your eyes in the opposite direction as you nod your head. Then move them in the same direction again. Alternate between those two combinations for a couple of times. Rest whenever you feel like it. Less is more.

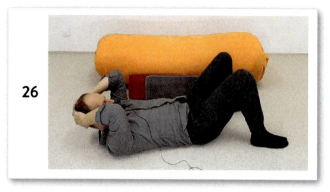

26

COMBINE: EYES, HEAD AND PELVIC MOVEMENTS

Now try to move your eyes, head, and pelvis into opposite directions, try various combinations. You will notice that looking up while lifting the head is easier than looking down while lifting the head. And that it is quite possible to learn to look in whichever direction you like – and still keep the same light quality of lifting the head. It's a big step forward in body control, freedom of movement, and awareness of self.

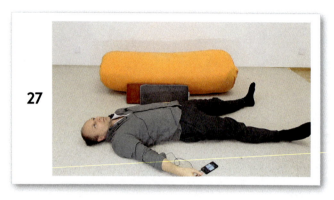

27

REST, SCAN, FEEL

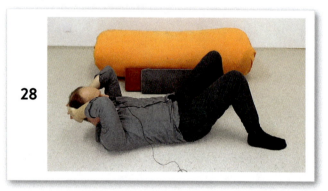

28

LIFT YOUR HEAD

Lift your head again in any way that comes to your mind, play a bit, be purposeful with a plan, and also try freestyle. Compare how it is now.

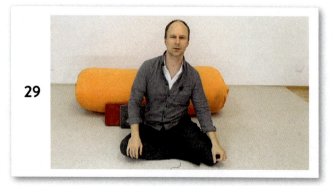

29

SIT UP

Come to sit. Feel how you carry the head. Move your head around a bit to see how it is. Combine your head movements with movements of your shoulder girdle, shoulders, torso, pelvis...

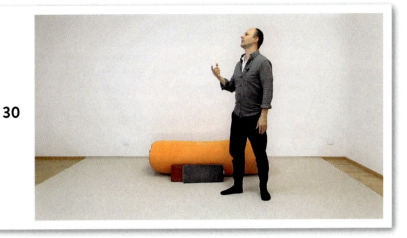

STAND UP
Come to standing, observe how you carry your head, your shoulders, your pelvis, how your weight is distributed over your feet...

 Specialisation IN A LIMITED RANGE OF ACTS FOR LONG PERIODS IS THE MOST DIFFICULT ADJUSTMENT —— FOR MAN TO MAKE. ——

If a man uses his eyes as people in the past did, i.e., to look at the horizon, at the sky, at his body and at his work, the eye goes through the complete range of its capacity, and ignorance of the proper use of the eyes has no chance to cause real harm. But when the scholar, or composer, or draughtsman has to use his eyes to focus at ten inches for hours on end, day after day, it is essential for him to know how to use the eyes properly. For he puts on them an extreme demand by excluding all functioning in favour of a particular act. Some muscles, nerves and cells in the higher centres are overworked, while others must be constantly inhibited. Only a few who thus use their eyes will succeed in preserving good use of them.

We often hear people say that their special incapacity is due to lack of exercise. Here we see that any training may be worse than no training at all; for the eyes of none of these people lack exercise, yet their eyesight deteriorates steadily. The use they make of their eyes adapts them most perfectly to that particular use only, but renders them almost useless for other purposes. Thus, even a young man with perfect eyesight will not see the details that a short-sighted histologist will see in his microscope. But whereas the former will rapidly adjust himself to the microscope, the latter is unable to get normal service from his eyes in any other use. In the same manner, any strong young man with perfect feet will find it difficult to stand as long as a flat-footed liftman, for instance, or policeman, but the former can jump and run, while the latter suffers aches and pains in doing so."

Quote from Dr. Moshé Feldenkrais, „Body and Mature Behaviour"

Ann Dyer Cervantes 1 month ago

Appreciate your teaching so much! I look forward to every new lesson.

StudioC98 4 days ago

Hi Alfons, thank you so much for your videos. As a classical pianist I can tell Feldenkrais has helped me to improve movements and flexibility a lot. I do go to classes but I practice with you at home or wherever I am :) I so appreciate your sense of humor and clarity. Greetings from NY! Laura

Skyler Shelton 11 months ago

Your videos are introducing me to Feldenkrais and I'm really grateful. You have a talent for instruction. I spend a lot of time on YT following tutorials and it's not typical for it to be such an enjoyable experience

Thanks for all the hard work you put into this!
Skyler in Arizona

Phil Gardner 1 year ago

My body felt like it was rocking on my hips at the end when standing - like the hip joints and vertebrae were so relaxed they didn't need to be tense to hold me upright. Very nice feeling - the Feldenkrais float. Thank you.

I also notice a stiffness in my lower and upper spine the morning after some of these lessons. It may be nothing to do with the lessons, but I suspect that the more I do Feldenkrais, the more my body releases old tensions as it re-adjusts to new ways of moving, and tensions that I would previously deal with through stretching, yoga or more more vigorous movements that I do each day. I may be wrong, but either way, I find it interesting.

Kevin Curtin 1 year ago

3rd day really is making that neck intercostal connection. Now that knee bend exercise where your eyes and chest move upwards as you rise become a lot clearer. The chest opening is really profound, and how it integrates with the neck and hips. Great stuff as usual. Kevin in Maine

alinaxek 2 months ago

Feeling wonderful ! Like after deep meditation. I found this video when seeking for Anit Baniel method about which I've read in the article about the harm of long sitting. But now I am your fan :). Thank you. I am from Lithuania.

florencia pina 7 months ago

this is brilliant!!! thank you,
florencia from santiago de Chile =)

allonespiriti 1 month ago

OMG. I am so grateful to Feldenkraise and you. Day 3 was a miracle for me. I have never been able to relax my left shoulder into the floor. I could never put both arms behind my head with elbows to sides- never in 45 years! I was only able to do a few of each lift and cannot touch or reach knee due to lower back injury. But I made the motion as if I could.

At the end of the wxercise I suddenly realized my left shoulder was lying on the bed with arms behind head. Something released that was holding the arm guarding my left side. Its miraculous. I am so grateful for you posting these. I have to do these on a firm bed as I cannot go to the floor- yet!

Thank you Alfons.

Ntathu Allen 1 year ago

Another day of feeling freer in my body. Thank you

Ed Sevensky 11 months ago

I like this new introductory series; well thought out and well presented. I have your book, but the visuals are a huge help.

Thanks for all the time you are devoting to this!

All testimonial citations in this chapter are from publicly visible comments in the public comment section of my YouTube video „IMPROVE POSTURE & CHEST FLEXIBILITY WITH THESE EASY MOVEMENTS", https://goo.gl/Zo3WR1, (December 4, 2017). I try to attribute as correctly as feasible, according to the official APA guidelines.

LESSON 3

Elbows towards knees

And what is good, Phaedrus,
— and what is not good —
need we ask anyone to tell us these things?

ROBERT M. PIRSIG

PLEASE WORK THROUGH THE VIDEO FIRST TO BENEFIT FULLY FROM THIS *Workbook*

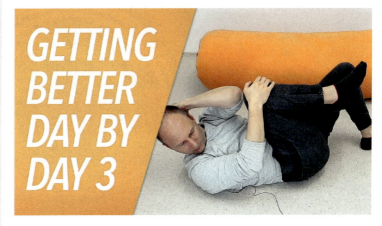

YOUTUBE VIDEO TITLE:
IMPROVE POSTURE & CHEST FLEXIBILITY WITH THESE EASY MOVEMENTS

The movements in this lesson seem to resemble the classic sit-up, and dangerously so. „Dangerously", because there's plenty of things that can go wrong with sit-ups (most prominently disc herniation). Gladly, we're not going to do this kind of abs strengthening exercise. We properly sliced this exercise to pieces, alas, re-built it from ground up, quite literally. The result is a

BEAUTIFUL

just beautiful FELDENKRAIS® movement sequence. And one of the most commonly taught lesson I guess, because it's so immensely beneficial. The previous two lessons beautifully led up to this one, and the following lessons will beautifully enhance and further build on it. So here's what's going to happen:

GRACEFUL

You will put to use everything you've learned so far in order to do a nice flexion movement in lying supine. You will gracefully distribute the flexion through your whole self, and eventually touch your elbows and knees together. You will become more flexible and at the same time better organised and better balanced. You will never stretch, never strain, and always stay within your comfort zone. How's that for „feldenkrais-ified"?

• •

ARRIVE ON THE FLOOR
Get on the floor and give yourself a minute or two to relax more fully to the floor. Briefly recap the previous lessons. Reduce the actual, bodily movements to such a tiny degree, that the movements only happen in your thinking. I call this „kinesthetic thinking".

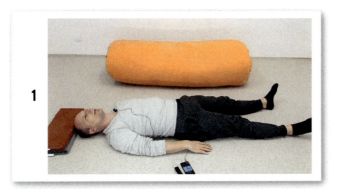

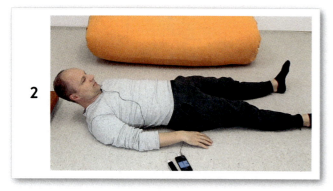

LIFT YOUR HEAD
With arms relaxed on the floor, lift your head a bit, a couple of times, to see how it is.

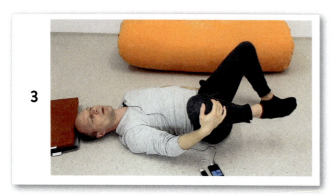

LINES AND CIRCLES WITH YOUR RIGHT KNEE
Hold you right knee with your right hand and casually and slowly explore some basic movements: Up, down, left, right, circles left and right. This, just as the „pelvic clock" is a classic FELDEN-KRAIS® movement combination. Be very aware of what is happening in your right hip joint and with your pelvis.

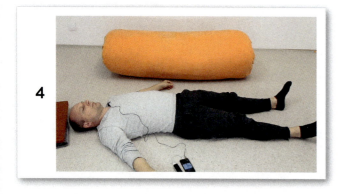

PAUSE

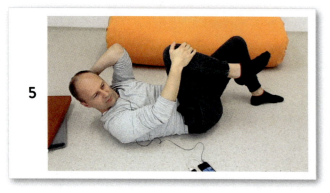

LEFT ELBOW TOWARDS RIGHT KNEE
Hold your head with your left hand. Start very small. Focus on the beginning of the movement. With each new movement make it a bit bigger. There's no need to touch the elbow to the knee. The journey is the reward.

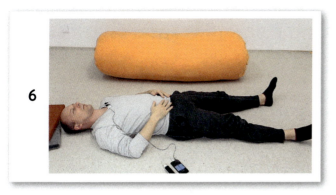

PAUSE

6

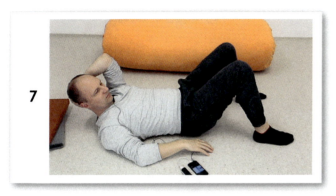

WITH YOUR LEFT HAND LIFT YOUR HEAD ALONG THE BODY MIDLINE

Hold your head with your left hand. Use your left hand to either completely support and carry your head or just move along with your head. Experiment with those two extremes. Lift your head along the midline of your torso.

7

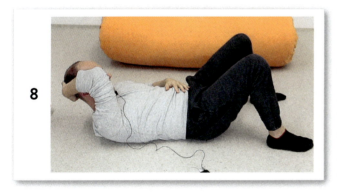

WITH YOUR RIGHT HAND LIFT YOUR HEAD ALONG THE BODY MIDLINE

This time use your right hand to help lift and guide your head. Try to lift exactly alongside the midline of your torso. How is that different from the previous movements? What does this demonstrate? We learn to move through movement, not through reading books.

8

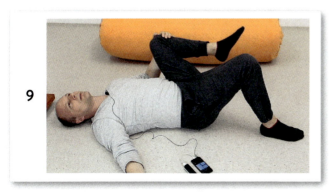

LINES AND CIRCLES WITH LEFT KNEE

Hold your left knee with your left hand and casually and slowly explore some basic movements: Up, down, left. right, circles left and right. Instead of focusing on the knee, explore the movements of your left hip joint, and how this connects to your pelvis. Does your pelvic roll? Or does it not move at all? What is happening? Why?

9

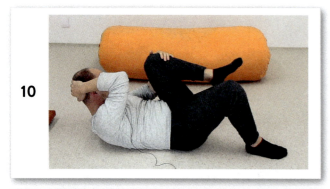

RIGHT ELBOW TOWARDS LEFT KNEE

Review all details: Lifting of the head, flexing of the spine, leaning against the floor, growing distance to the floor, shifting point of contact to the floor, rolling of the pelvis, breathing, using your eyes to direct movement... what else?

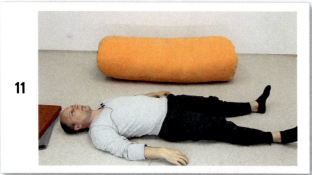

PAUSE

Explore the difference between thinking about a movement, and thinking a movement, and actually moving. Think about how small you can do a movement. What's the slowest and smallest way to move?

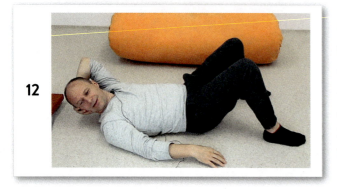

LIFT HEAD – FACING RIGHT

Turn your head to the right, place your head into the palm of your left hand. Do not crack your neck – this is not for chiropractic adjustment. Gently and carefully start lifting your head. What can you learn in this variation? How is this different to before?

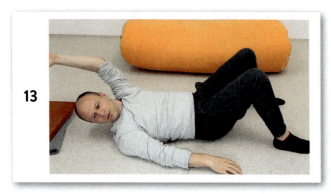

LIFT YOUR HEAD WITH YOUR LEFT ARM STRAIGHT OVERHEAD

Keep your head turned to the right. The starting position is with your left arm extended (if possible), resting on the floor (if possible), over your head, in extension of your spine so to speak, with your head turned to the right. Lift your head and arm together. Do this many times. After each movement start from scratch. Change how much you do. Change how fast you lift. Explore slightly different alignments.

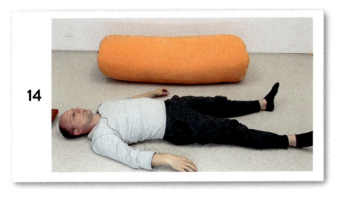

PAUSE

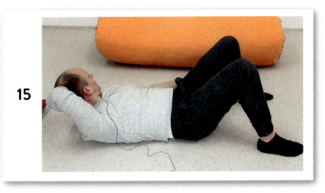

LIFT YOUR HEAD – FACE LEFT

This time rest your left cheek (or left ear) in your right hand. Lift your head like before. Try to make it smooth.

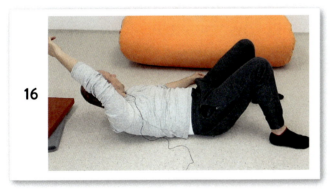

LIFT YOUR HEAD WITH YOUR RIGHT ARM STRAIGHT OVERHEAD

Keep your head turned to the left. Your right arm is extended upwards. Not towards the ceiling, but upwards in the direction of your head. When you are resting your straight right arm (if possible) is lying on the floor (if possible). Do not strain. Think approximations.

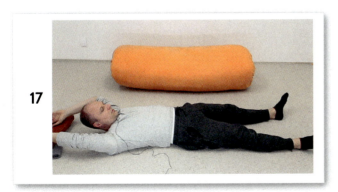

LIFT HEAD WITH BOTH ARMS STRAIGHT ON THE FLOOR

Don't take shortcuts. Don't rush. Lift your head without lifting your arms. Give your full attention to each new movement. Immerse yourself in the process. Be the process.

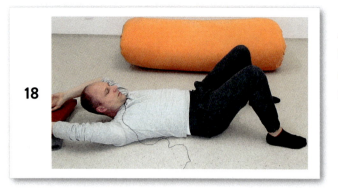

AGAIN, BUT WITH FEET STANDING
Lift your head with both arms straight overhead on the floor, but this time with your feet standing. How is this different?

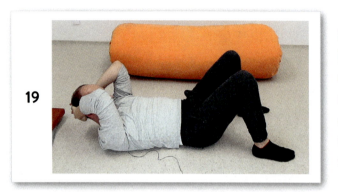

USE YOUR HANDS TO LIFT YOUR HEAD, SCAN, COMPARE
Compare to the beginning of the lesson. How have the movements changed? How has your thinking and perception changed? Your ability to feel? Your understanding of these movements and your ability to verbalize what is happening?

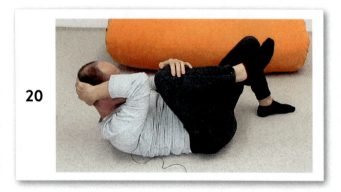

RIGHT ELBOW TOWARDS RIGHT KNEE
The objective is not to touch, but to move them towards each other. You can touch them together though, if you like. But it's neither an requirement nor the goal.

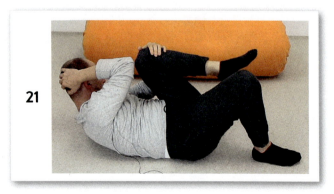

RIGHT ELBOW TOWARDS LEFT KNEE
This is a slightly different trajectory than the previous move. What are the differences? Can you sense the differences?

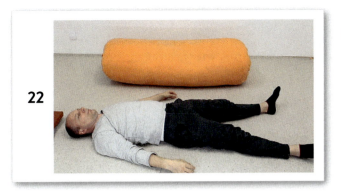

PAUSE

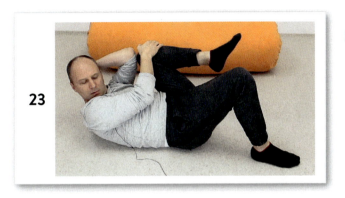

LEFT ELBOW TOWARDS LEFT KNEE

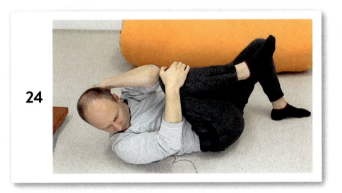

LEFT ELBOW TOWARDS RIGHT KNEE

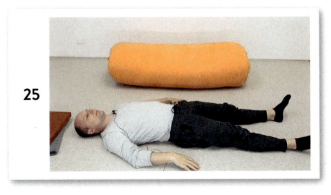

TAKE A GOOD REST
Feel how resting feels now. Review the last four movements in kinesthetic thinking. They have been quite similar, but also quite different. „Same same but different", so they say.

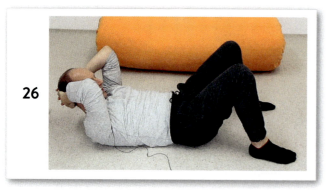

LIFT YOUR HEAD
Wrap it up, try lifting your head again, a bit. This is our reference movement. We use this movement to notice changes to how it was and how it is now. You can use this movement once in a while to check where you're at. And if you should work through this lesson again.

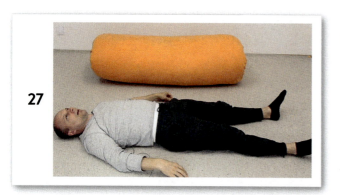

PAUSE

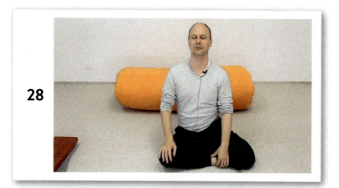

SIT UP
Come to sit, feel how you carry the head

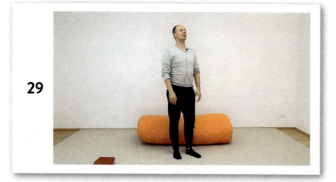

STAND UP
Come to stand, observe how you carry your head, your shoulders, your pelvis (what?), your weight distribution over your feet, on your feet…

kirsten menzel 7 months ago

This lesson is amazing. At the end when I stranded I felt really erecting with no effort, and with and especial feeling into my body like a springs. Walk was very funny and easy, some kind of a dance

dominette 8 months ago

This was awesome..you are so funny..I have great laughs. My body has never felt better. The past couple of days I have been doing some heavy garden work..I woke up much to my surprise with NO back pain..I attribute this to Feldenkrais. I have been doing the core work, and many of the other classes with you. Going to go through ask of these classes.

I am thrilled...out here in beautiful Austin Texas.

I went through Austria as a teenager/musician on the road..It is so beautiful. Through the Brenner Pass in the height of winter with no heat in an old Volkswagen bus. Thank you so so so much.

Fran Sharpe 1 month ago

Thanks for a lovely lesson. I like the way you enjoy playing with the English language, too!

Penthesilea 2 months ago

You mentioned taking a half moment to relax and refresh ... I am retired and I live alone so my time is 100% my own. I am so grateful that I found your channel. I am taking my time to luxuriate into these movements. How lucky am I? Thank you for this precious gift of helping me flow into body nirvana.

TT 1 year ago

Thank you so much for taking the time to make and share these lessons. Looking forward to the next lesson :)

Joy Greenhalgh 2 months ago

Greetings from England ! This brings happiness to my body and so to my mind. Thank you Alfons !

Julie Sager 1 year ago

As always, Alfons, excellent lesson! I appreciate your expertise in the Feldenkrais Method. Thank you, Julie in Colorado

kira mango 9 months ago

Hi Alfons. So, I've hit a sort of wall here. When I do this one I feel worse particularly in the groin/tops of thighs around hip joint, where there is pain anyway. Have tried doing less, but there is something about going in that direction - forward towards knees - that irritates what is already going on. Any suggestions?

AND Thank You for you great work on these Youtube videos and making this available to those of us out in the hinterlands!

pezchi 4 months ago

Aged 80, I am a great believer in the Feldenkrais method. The movements are always gentle, always slow and an efficient way to keep the body supple, flexible and pain free.

Could I please, suggest an arm movement when in any of the resting periods. Try this - rest your arms on the floor above your head. At first, it maybe difficult but keep trying and you will succeed. All babies lie like this when on their back and somehow as adults we lose the feeling of comfort with this arm position, which is a pity. This position is good because it opens up the chest, the lungs and the breath while resting.

Thank you Alfons for your very nice lessons.

KL Power 1 year ago

I am feeling the results of these movement in enhanced relaxation and flexibility, and in soreness of muscles used. For example, I never knew how heavy my head was until I tried to lift it with one hand. Thank you, Alfons.

Elizabeth Kurjata 1 year ago

Constantly recommend my clients sign up with you! You make this fun!

Lynn McCoy Sloan 4 weeks ago

Feldenkrais is completely new to me. I decided to take a youtube look into it after The NYTimes published an article on Feldenkrais last week. And here I am in your daily lessons. I love the idea of 'making peace with gravity' and getting to know the intimate relationship with my skeletal system. Such a wonderful missing link for me as I strive to be healthy mainly through restorative yoga and gentle swimming. I plan on revisiting this lesson in particular. A good start for the release my shoulders/neck have been craving for years. Thank you!!!

Anth8787 7 months ago

Alfons- I have done many of your video lessons. This is my 2nd time doing your 10 - video series, and I intend to use your hip workshop to teach myself to walk properly again. I will continue comment through my journey. Thank you for sharing yourself and allowing me to participate in your passion.

Jin Jandovitz 1 year ago

Hi Dear, I love this title, I am "Getting better day by day" , thank you very much. I don't remember which video you talked about -- make an attempt to move but not really moving, I follow this concept when I lying down or even on the train, I felt my breathing pattern is changing and found alignment on the spot. I even found my 3rd eye easily by pretending to open my eyes in my Kundalini yoga class. :)

5vaVinia5 6 months ago

Hi Alfons. I want to say THANK YOU!!! for the wonderful contribution you are making with these lessons. All the ones I have tried already are giving me a great improvement to my body. This one in particular has been great for my shoulders and flexibility in my neck. Thanks again!!!

Charlotte Wilson 4 months ago

Thank you, there was much freedom for my neck and shoulders. I am gaining so much from your videos. I like your teaching style. I bought your kindle book but prefer following the videos for now.
I'm a yoga teacher.

Doris Hasslocher 11 months ago

Thank you!! I have done this same lesson several times before, from other sources, and while I always liked it and got some benefit, I have never had such a sudden and dramatic benefit until I did yours today! I know the purists think you shouldn't demonstrate Feldenkrais, but it makes such a difference to be able to see that it is possible to do it faster, or slower or bigger or smaller or with more bending, or whatever, than what I could come up with by myself. I had always kept my elbows more stiff and not wanted to move my torso because I somehow thought I wasn't supposed to, even though nobody said I wasn't supposed to, then I saw you do the movement with so much more aliveness, and so I got some of your aliveness into my movement, instead of my robotness, and it made a HUGE difference!!! You are my new Feldenkrais hero and I'm so glad I found you!

doristea 4 months ago

Dear Alfons this lesson makes me realize and relief my chest issues. At the end my chest feels free and pirouettes. Thank you so much. Regards

Leah Twitchell 1 year ago

My shoulders are so happy with this lesson! They were previously abused with too much yoga asana and P90x, so it's time to give them some love. :) This whole series has been amazing. My body is naturally holding itself in a better posture. For example, I can feel my scapulae are now more flat on my back (less winging). Thank you so much! :)

T π 1 year ago

Very interesting lesson, thank you... My elbow "medial epicondyle" got very sore & irritated from the pressure of them on the floor while moving my arms. I will repeat this lesson again, next time I'll use a blanket under my arms.

All testimonial citations in this chapter are from publicly visible comments in the public comment section of my YouTube video „RELAX SHOULDERS & IMPROVE HEAD TURN", https://goo.gl/ztjCj3, (December 5, 2017). I try to attribute as correctly as feasible, according to the official APA guidelines.

LESSON 4

Getting to know the shoulder girdle and its connections to the whole body

What would the world be like without Captain Hook?

CAPTAIN HOOK

PLEASE WORK THROUGH THE
VIDEO FIRST
TO BENEFIT FULLY FROM THIS
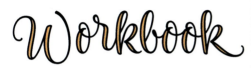

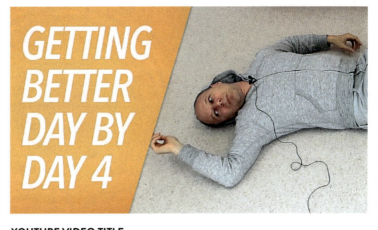

YOUTUBE VIDEO TITLE:
RELAX SHOULDERS & IMPROVE HEAD TURN

You will get to know your shoulder girdle in great detail. You will explore how the movements of your shoulder blades relate to the movements of your arms, and how your neck has to respond.

RE-DISCOVER

You will discover order and meaning in a seemingly endless range of random possibilities and combinations. Re-discovering your shoulder girdle and its wide spread connections will make you feel refreshed, alive and in-the-know.

RE-ORGANIZE

I recommend to introduce a short rest in between every step. Maybe even a mini nap here or there. Or a break. Go get a glass of water or something, put your laundry into the washing machine, update your facebook status, then continue. I feel this is a very demanding lesson which might lead to a powerful re-organization of your shoulder girdle and its connection to various areas of your body. Take your time, maybe start over again, take a lot of rests, pauses, breaks. Here we go:

ARRIVE ON THE FLOOR

Get on the floor and give yourself a minute or two until you can't relax any further. In FELDENKRAIS® lessons you are the center of your world, and thus you have to look at the relative directions accordingly. In lying supine **IN FRONT** is where the ceiling is, **UP** is in the direction of your head, **DOWN** is in the direction of your feet, **BEHIND** is where the floor is. In other words: „forwards" and „upwards" are not the same. But which one is which?

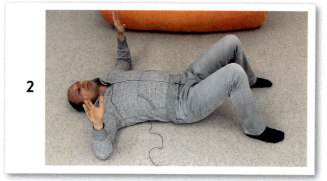

GET INTO THE STARTING POSITION

Upper arms in (preferably exactly) 90 degrees angle in relation to your torso. Lower arms standing on elbows, in a 90 degree angle to your upper arm. To keep this 90-90 constraint is SUPER IMPORTANT. Otherwise there's little to no connection to the lower, floating ribs. Feet should be standing, knees pointing towards the ceiling. The rest can go (and move) wherever you want.

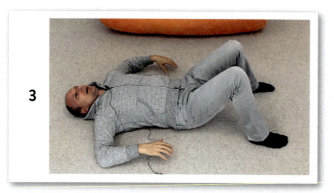

LOWER HANDS DOWNWARDS

Bring palms towards floor. DO NOT change the 90 degree angles. Check frequently to make sure the 90 degrees are still there. Never strain, do not stretch, stay within your comfort zone.

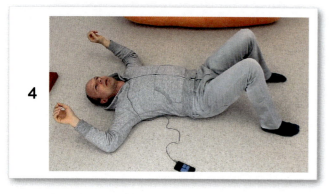

RAISE HANDS UPWARDS

Bring the back of your hands towards the floor. Do not move or slide your elbows. Your elbows should stay in place. Keep the 90 degree angle at all costs. Even if that means that you can't touch the floor with your fingers.

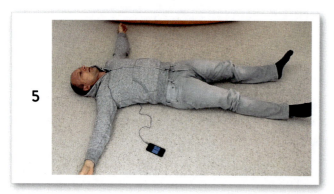

HAVE A BREAK

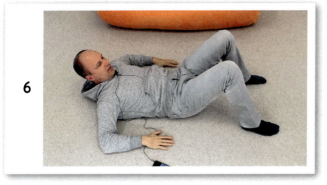

6

LOWER HANDS DOWNWARDS AND LIFT HEAD AND SHOULDERS

Same as before [3], but also lift your head & shoulders. Feel your shoulder blades slide up and around. Your front side becoming shorter, your back side becoming longer. You (should) know that move from the previous lessons.

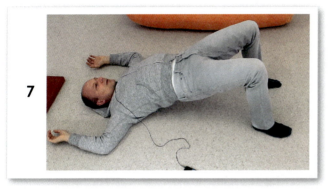

7

RAISE HANDS UPWARDS AND LIFT YOUR PELVIS

Same as before [4], but also lift your pelvis. Feel your shoulder blades slide town towards your buttocks and your spine. Coordinate your arm–head–neck–shoulder movements, experiment with what „part" moves first („movement initiation"), how you synchronize movements etc.

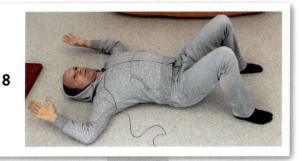

8

COMBINE: HANDS UPWARDS AND DOWNWARDS

Compare how the previous movements [3] + [4] have changed. How do you feel and what can you observe now? Combine those two movements. It's your life, your body, your time. As a teacher I'm not controlling you, I'm not observing you, you're not under surveillance. Play a bit with those movements and movement combinations. They do matter. They are part of a sequence. There is enough order in the sequence for you to get creative and play with it. But be careful, gentle, love your moves, don't hurt yourself.

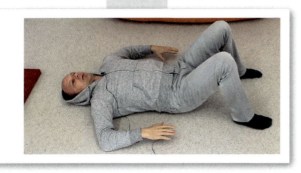

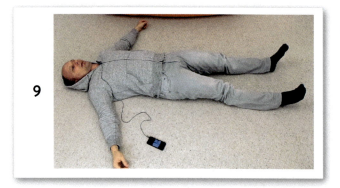

REST

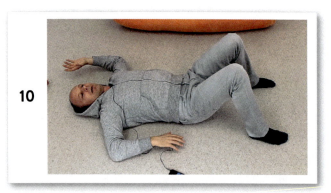

HANDS IN OPPOSITE DIRECTIONS

Move one hand upwards, while you move the other one downwards. Feel the opposite rotation in your upper arms. Alternate. Make sure to keep the 90-90 angles.

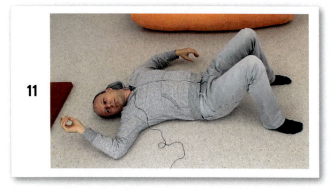

LET YOUR HEAD ROLL

Continue with the previous arm movements, but let go of your neck muscles. In which direction does your head roll? Do not roll your head deliberately. Let it roll as a consequence of your arm movements.

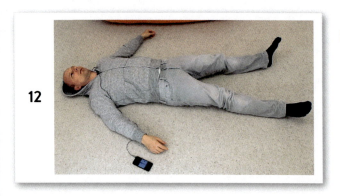

REST

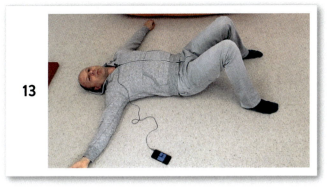

ROLL YOUR FISTS

Start with your arms in a 90 degree angle to the torso, with elbows extended. Make fists (more or less), start rolling one arm upwards while you roll the other one downwards. In PT language it's called internal and external humeral rotation. Also think of rolling your fists. Keep as close as feasible to the 90 degree angles.

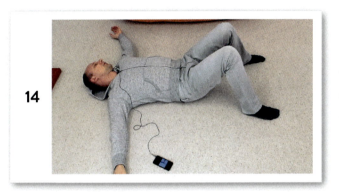

LET YOUR HEAD ROLL

Don't clench your teeth or jaw, don't hold your breath. Rotate and roll your fists in opposite directions and let your head roll. Don't make it happen, instead let it happen.

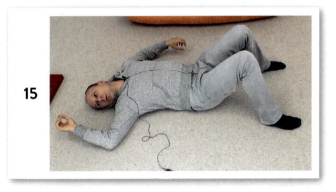

HANDS UPWARDS AND DOWNWARDS

With 90-90 degrees arms, move one hand upwards and one hand downwards, that is hands in opposite directions, let your head roll. See how it is compared to before [11].

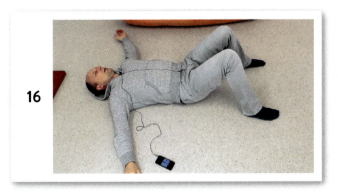

FLEX AND EXTEND ELBOWS WHILE ROLLING

Continue the previous movement [15], but alternate between extended and 90-90 degree flexed elbows. In other words: keep your arms on the floor. You might need a Camebridge-MIT degree of Movement Sciences to be able to accomplish this ;-)

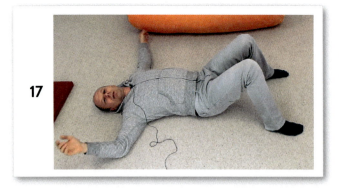

FREESTYLE
Continue, play with various degrees of extension and flexion of your elbows.

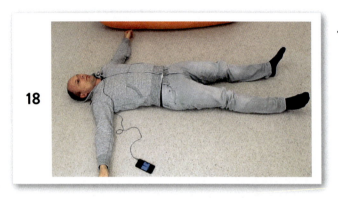

TAKE A REST

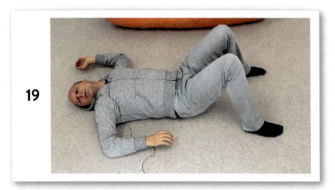

HEAD IN „WRONG" DIRECTION
Return to the previous 90-90 movement [15]: With 90-90 degrees arms, move one hand upwards and one hand downwards, that is hands in opposite directions, let your head roll. However, this time, roll your head in the „wrong" direction, in the direction where your hand is going down. Make sure to keep your 90-90 degree angles.

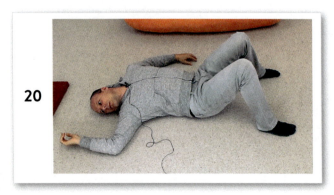

HANDS UPWARDS AND DOWNWARDS
Return to the 90-90 movement, turn your head in the direction where the hand is going up. See how it is now. Change between the previous [19] and this movement and see how they affect each other. Every time you change between these two variations the other variation will become smoother, easier, more of a second nature.

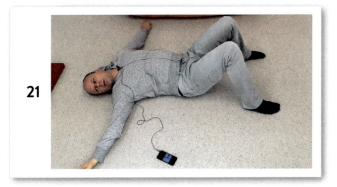

21

ROLL ARMS ON FLOOR

Roll your arms on the floor. Observe how it is now. Let your whole self participate.

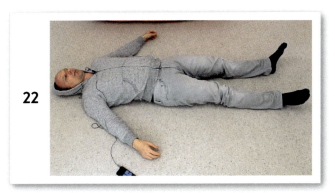

22

REST

Take one last rest to observe yourself and your contact to the floor. Use the floor as a reference to inquire about the state your shoulders are in and how you are resting.

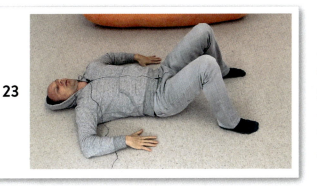

23

REFERENCE MOVEMENT: MOVE HANDS DOWN

Get into the 90-90 degree starting position with your feet standing and hands towards the ceiling as in [2], and then move your hands downwards towards the floor. How is it now? How is it different to the beginning?

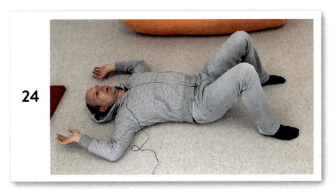

24

REFERENCE MOVEMENT: MOVE HANDS UP

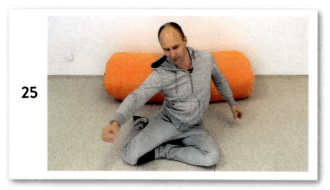

SIT UP

Observe yourself in sitting

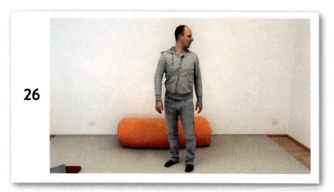

STAND UP

Observe yourself in standing, try how movement works for you now. Turn your head around, it may have improved significantly.

Alice Aird 1 month ago

Thank you so much for this interesting and effective lesson Alfons! I have had immediate and enormous benefit after only doing it once, then again today two days later, I have received similar improvement. My shoulders, even my sore left one, move so freely and it's a pleasure to feel the difference.
I have a very sore left shoulder with damage to tendons, as I'm told by doctors. It didn't seem to improve at all until I did this lesson no matter what else I tried. Thank you thank you thank you!

Pippi DiMerlo 7 months ago

Hi Alfons, by the end of the lesson touching both palms to the floor was EASY. Fantastic! Thank you.

Jonatan Bogren 1 year ago

Like it! Very interesting exploring in this manner.. I was intrigued by Feldenkrain after reading the brain that heals itself by Norman Doidge

Claire Pickin 7 months ago

My favourite lesson so far Alfons - discovered some new things about my shoulders! I felt like I had new shoulders by the end of the session! Thank you!

Natala 9 1 month ago

Never have I been so aware of my shoulder blades relative to shoulder-arm movement.
Thank you as always!

Peri Miller 1 year ago

Thanks so much Alfons! I have really enjoyed your videos! I like this new series that you have started. I completed this video with the most incredible shoulder opening. I had a real 'aha moment' when you directed us to do the same movement with the arms extended with loose fists. After that point my shoulders relaxed even more. Thanks again I look forward to all your upcoming videos.

alinaxek 2 months ago

Thanks Alfons, I.ve experienced another wonderful lesson! I have some shoulder problems. When I was rolling extended arms for the first time I felt pain in my left shoulder but when this was done after several minutes - there was no pain! When lying on the floor at the end of the lesson, I feel the left side ribs more on the floor than the right side.

J Algar 1 year ago

Alfons, I cannot thank you enough! I enjoy your teaching style, both with your playful humour and patient explanation. I have learned to much and your teachings have helped me immensely!!
I live in Canada, so being able to watch, learn and participate with your videos is a blessings. You are such an amazing person. This video, in particular, gave me so much insight as to how tight and restricted my shoulders were ... and how relaxed and mobile they became.

dominette 8 months ago

such an amazing feeling, thank you.

pedanticmofo 2 months ago

At the beginning of this lesson, it was a lot harder to rotate my right arm forward and my left arm back. Maybe a little less so after, but the lesson left me feeling very twisted up. I looked in the mirror and my hips had shifted several inches to the left and my right shoulder had dropped several inches below the right. I also noticed that my right knee kept falling inward. No pain, not that I had any before, and my neck and upper back are more free-moving, but the result feels really awkward.

Hafdis Lilja Pétursdóttir 9 months ago

Óskaplega eru þetta góðar æfingar fyrir mig. Elska þær, bestu þakkir.

George Hudacko 11 months ago

Really enjoying the results and your delivery. Plus love your 'impishness' Sweet flavoring in your German accent, Geo.

Linda Cantor 4 months ago

I am 80 years old, and find these lessons free my body beautifully. They help me be more conscious of my movements and beginning to make adjustments throughout the day. I am very thankful for your presentation with playfulness as it reminds me to be more playful also.

Phil Gardner 1 year ago

Yes, definitely a snug fit with the floor at the end and a freeing of the shoulders and upper body. My neck is quite long and I've often had tension there (partly due to old injuries), so there was a bit of clicking in the vertebrae at the end, but I assume this is normal due to re-organising joints and bones.
I liked the lesson a lot.

Ετέαρχος Κατσούγκρης 10 months ago

we love it...

Elizabeth Suhr 2 months ago

Thanks Alfons, your lessons are wonderful - engaging, playful and enlightening! I have such longstanding tightness throughout my body from poor postural patterns that I'm unable to lift my head off the floor without feeling a lot of tension and strong discomfort through my neck, shoulders chest and upper back, but I'm hopeful that this will improve with time and I'm finding your videos very helpful

Sanne vd Horst 7 months ago

Wunderbar indeed ;-) Loving ure introduction in Feldenkrais [..] Funny, at the age of 46, learning about my own bones and how they work. Thank u for the beginners lessons! And ure humor, makes it even fun to watch as well!!

Sadhana Yoga 10 months ago

Thank you Alfons. Lovely natural delivery. And very enjoyable & effective. I look forard to more. L

Ntathu Allen 1 year ago

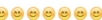

Penthesilea 2 months ago

Immediately upon sitting up, my upper right side felt beautifully relaxed and light. This is the side that has been tormenting me for 50 years. When I lifted my right arm it felt like a cloud. My left side, which usually feels pretty good, felt like a bucket of rusty, decrepit bones and bolts. So I immediately restarted the video, laid back down and treated my left side to this beautiful lesson. Thank you, Maestro.

Natala 9 1 month ago

This was so relaxing that I kept falling asleep, just like in Bell Hand. Your skeletal intro, however, and attention to wrist and upward left my wrist and even my shoulder feeling looser and more free. Will definitely do this on the other side.

Sanne vd Horst 7 months ago

What a difference in both sides of the body now! I'm gonna find some time soon to work with the other hand! Thank u!

Julie Fitzgerald 1 year ago

I didn't expect my right leg, which usually feels shorter than my left, to feel longer and my foot to feel very relaxed in standing after this lesson. Wow!

L. Hulsizer 9 months ago

Fabulous. I have had a swimmer's shoulder... this really helped. Thank you.

Gyan S. Tomasic 7 months ago

Hello Alfons, thank you for this video. It is deemed most worthy, enabling many of us to reclaim the ally of our right and left arm. A nice feeling to have the arms float upwards towards the ceiling. I especially felt a great benefit thumping the left shoulder blade down on the floor, particularly since both shoulder blades had previously been locked in and down to a limited range of immobility (due to condition that I had been diagnosed with), and over time loosening the shoulder blades. I so enjoy your lessons and your good humour and how you use the English language.... it is a bit odd when one looks at the words. hahahaha. Many thanks.

1990Abbadon 1 year ago

thx for the great lesson! it's always funny to see one shoulder hanging much lower than the other after a one-sided feldenkrais lesson.

M Kay 11 months ago

Thank you, thank you, thank you Alfons! Such a gift to give everyone. There is no feldenkrais classes in my area and I have long been interested so I thank you so very much. Internal body awareness is so important. We just take for granted and abuse ourselves. I am learning to "micro listen" to my body...it feels like it is starting to float. :) When I focus just on the micro movements my mind becomes still and calm. I use is as part of my Meditation and I am loving it. With love.

Lolo 1 year ago

Thank you very much for your lovely lessons Alfons, I've had tendonitis in my right shoulder for over 10 years and these feldenkrais videos are helping me with my healing incredibly. Especially the learning how to relax through movement part. I had a particularly rough day and then this lovely lesson conveniently popped up for me :) Your instructions are clear and your channel is great! My gratitude for all the awesome free content! I'll keep an eye out for updates from you

Mary B-P 7 months ago

I love this lesson Alfons, I play the piano, and my practice felt so much more natural & enjoyable.. more ease & connection! Thankyou

Miruna Macavei 10 months ago

Thank you for this lesson, Alfons! My right arm is now big, heavy and relaxed and I feel less of a tension headache that I've been having.

Olga Shmidov 1 year ago

Dear Alfons. What s a great lesson!!!! My right shoulder feels so better!!!! [..] Thank you soooo much..
Olga

All testimonial citations in this chapter are from publicly visible comments in the public comment section of my YouTube video „WRIST PAIN, CARPAL TUNNEL, FROZEN SHOULDER?", https://goo.gl/dRqad7, (December 5, 2017). I try to attribute as correctly as feasible, according to the official APA guidelines.

LESSON 5

Floating & lengthening, starting with your dominant hand

The hand is the dearest thing.
They know to do things with it.

MOSHÉ FELDENKRAIS

PLEASE WORK THROUGH THE **VIDEO FIRST** **TO BENEFIT FULLY FROM THIS**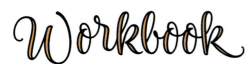

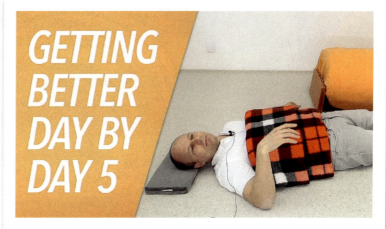

YOUTUBE VIDEO TITLE:
WRIST PAIN, CARPAL TUNNEL, FROZEN SHOULDER?

This lesson, like every lesson, serves several purposes. Most prominently it helps with the maintenance of your hands, most dominantly with your active AKA dominant hand: to remove unnecessary tension, to make it softer, more comfortable, get relief from sore areas or help stiff fingers become less troublesome. Dr. Moshé Feldenkrais said to his students: „The active, dominant hand of everyone is too strained. Of everyone, without exception. With everyone it interferes with breathing. With everyone it shortens the spine."

RELEASE

Furthermore this lesson teaches you how releasing tension in your hand might also release tension in your neck. If you have pain in the left arm or the left side of the neck, use your left hand. Everything is connected. Of course, if you work with your left side, you will need to translate what is written to the left side. You may very well repeat this lesson several times though, on either side.

SPREAD OUT

This lesson will help you to refine movement quality, to improve how your fingers relate to each other and spread out in relaxation, and it will help you to better understand your hand movements in general. It will make you become more aware of the various soft limits of movement and also the possibilities. This takes time. Make sure you're comfortable and undisturbed. When you do this lesson for the first time you might want to start with your dominant hand (the hand you use for writing, eating, brushing your teeth).

LIGHTNESS

This lesson also teaches how to move without shortening yourself. And how to avoid unnecessary effort in areas such as your neck, jaw, spine and your breathing. In fact, legend has it, that some people grew to be up to one inch taller with the help of this lesson. When getting up from the floor it teaches you to float up rather than to ache and muscle your way up. In this sense you will experience a whole new movement quality, movement organisation, and an overall pleasant sensation of ease and lightness.

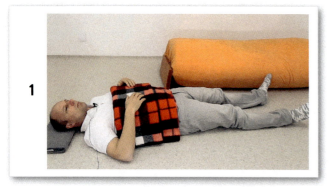

ARRIVE ON THE FLOOR
Get comfortable on the floor. Maybe take a cosy blanket to keep yourself warm. Stand your feet or rest your legs straight, it's up to you.

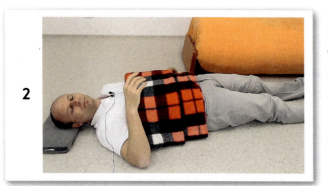

STAND YOUR LOWER ARM
This is the starting position from which we will start most of the moves. Keep your lower arm erect like a tower, or candle; not slanted like the leaning tower of Pisa, or a drawbridge of a medieval castle. Your hand should be standing directly over your elbow.

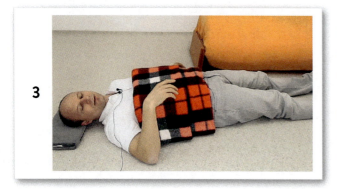

LET YOUR HAND SINK OVER
Let your hand gradually fall over towards the side of your palm. Slowly. Like it's sinking in driftsand. A palmar flexion without the effort. Let your hand loosen in the wrist to let it sink over in slow motion, and then slowly, slowly erect it. You will notice many things that you did not know before – IF you start doing this truly slowly. The quality of how you move, as well as the speed, makes or breaks this lesson.

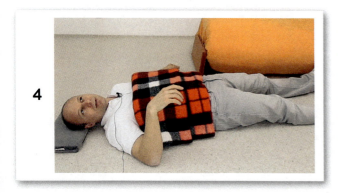

OBSERVE YOUR FINGERS
Observe the pathways your fingers take while you let your hand sink. Keep your lower arm straight up, standing at all times. In this context „observe" doesn't necessarily mean „to look" but rather to feel, to sense, to notice, to know.

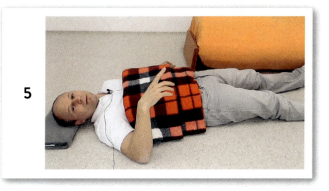

MOVE YOUR INDEX FINGER ONLY

Feel the pathway of your index finger. It's not a wiggling movement. It's not active flexion and active extension. It's flexion and let go again. Or extension and let go again. Or, yes, maybe also a combination of those two. You can let your index finger direct the movement of your entire hand.

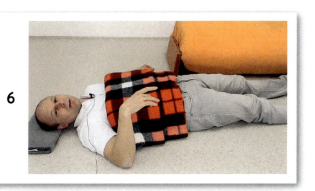

MOVE YOUR MIDDLE FINGER ONLY

It's quite difficult to inhibit the movement of the other fingers. Try small and slow movements. Lift or lower the middle finger just a tiny little bit at first, and with every move make it bigger.

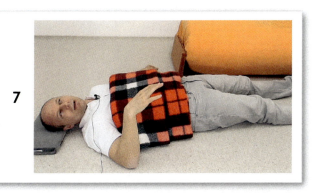

MOVE YOUR RING FINGER ONLY

Do not jiggle your finger, but think, lift, sink, feel, explore. Instead of forcing this finger to move separately from the other fingers, try to bring your awareness to your ring finger. It's about awareness and not execution to perfection. Don't force it.

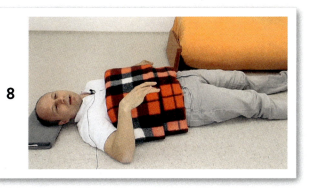

PINKY FINGER ONLY

Explore the same things with your pinky finger. You will also notice that little by little you can let the fingers direct the movement of your entire hand. Don't do any awkward contortions, just find what feels good and natural.

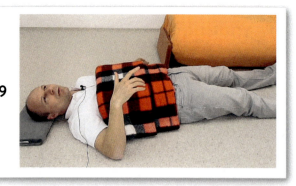

MOVE YOUR THUMB ONLY

The opposing thumb. Its movement pathways feel quite different to those of the other fingers, don't they?

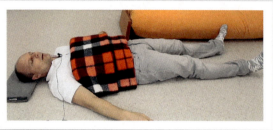

TAKE A REST

Short pause, rest, and feel how your arm is resting, how your fingers are resting.

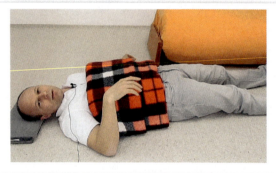

LET YOUR HAND SINK OVER

Compare how it is to the beginning of the lesson [3].

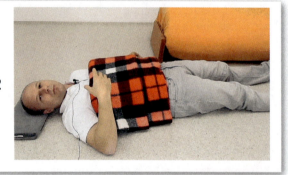

ROTATE YOUR LOWER ARM

Let your hand hang while you rotate your lower arm. Find the easy range, the soft and the hard limits, try to move homogeneously, same speed everywhere, move slowly.

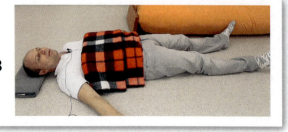

TAKE A REST

Pay attention if there was any unnecessary tension while you practiced, somewhere in your arm, or even your neck, eyes, shoulders, in your breathing.

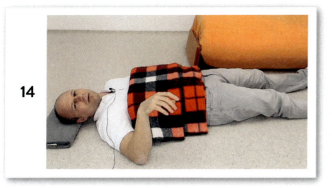

14

LET YOUR HAND SINK OVER, WITH HAND TURNED OUTWARDS

Point your relaxed fingers outwards, away from your chest, as far as possible without strain. In this position lift and sink your hand. Let each of your fingers move along it's own pathway. Observe, rather than direct.

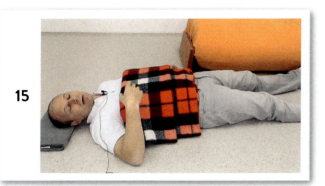

15

LET YOUR HAND SINK OVER, WITH HAND TURNED INWARDS

Point your relaxed fingers inwards, towards your face or chest, as far as possible without strain. Lift and sink your hand in this position.

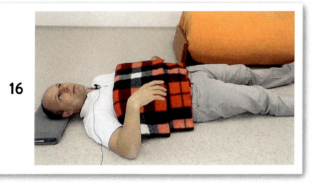

16

ROTATE LOWER ARM

Compare how it is now to how it was before [12].

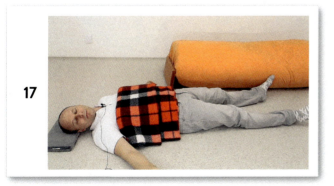

17

TAKE A REST

Compare to how you rested before. Is your arm more at ease, resting more clearly, thoroughly? How about your whole self?

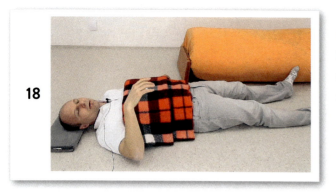

LIFT ELBOW A LITTLE BIT
Lift your elbow a tiny little bit off the floor, think of floating, levitating, or a breeze of wind pushing it away from the floor.

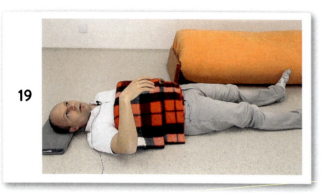

FIND THE BEST PATHWAY TO LIFT
Lift your elbow as before, do not interfere with your breathing. Try to have a „long" spine. Try not to shorten yourself. Let your lower arm, your elbow, your entire arm, float upwards. Find the path of least resistance.

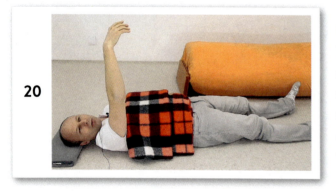

LIFT ELBOW FURTHER AWAY FROM THE FLOOR
Continue floating up your elbow until you can extend your arm easily, with seemingly no effort. Be aware of the pathway. Don't go down the dark path of muscling your arm up. Tempting it is, forever will it dominate your destiny, consume you it will.

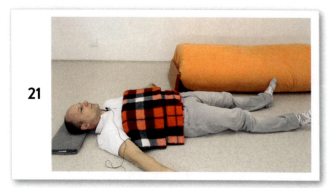

TAKE A BREAK
Rest for just a second or so, but stop the lesson and then start again. Take it as an opportunity to lose the new found movement quality and then find it again.

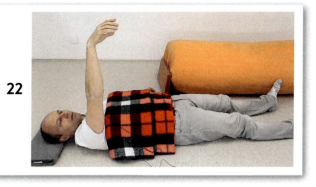

LIFT YOUR HAND

Float your elbow again, think of your hand floating away from the floor towards the ceiling. Find the same quality of movement again. Do not clench your teeth, do not tighten your neck muscles or chest. Do not interfere with your breathing. Do not shorten yourself.

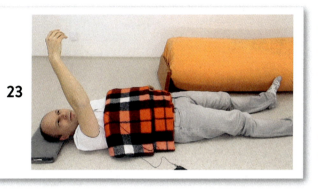

LET YOUR ARM SWAY UPWARDS AND DOWNWARDS

Arm extended, in an upright position. Remember: upwards and downwards is different to forwards and backwards. While swaying your arm upwards towards your head, and downwards towards your feet, let your arm rotate however much it wants.

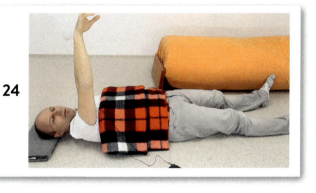

LIFT YOUR ARM

Start with your arm extended. Instead of floating your elbow, float your straight arm up. Maybe think of your shoulder blade. Then let your vertical arm sink back to stand on the floor again. Use the same movement quality as before when lifting the elbow.

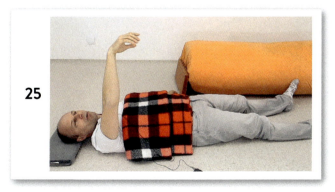

STOMP YOUR SHOULDER BLADE

After lifting your arm, let your straight arm fall towards the floor, it's like your stomping the floor, but with your shoulder blade instead of your foot. Or maybe think of knocking on the floor with a broom stick.

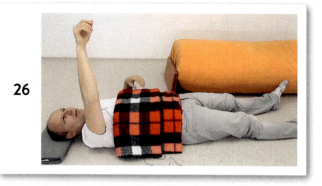

STOMP FASTER
Pick up speed. Faster and faster, until the point of contact between your shoulder blade and the floor becomes obvious. Where is it exactly? ... pam pam pam

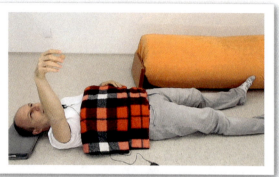

SWAYING ARM MOVEMENTS
Arm extended, standing. Left, right, upwards, downwards. Become more aware of where your arm is standing on the floor, how your arm can rotate while swaying. Relaxed hand with fingers hanging.

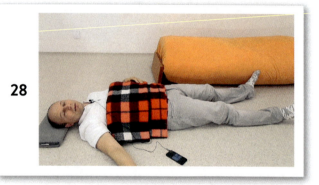

FLOAT DOWN, PAUSE
Let your arm float down again, take a rest

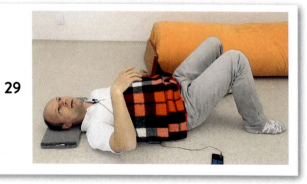

REVIEW
Review the whole floating sequence step by step.
Float your elbow up a couple of times more.
Let yourself be relaxed.
Don't let tension come into your body while lifting your elbow. Don't hold your breath, don't tighten your chest, don't clench your teeth.
Keep your spine long.
Float your elbow until your arm is fairly straight.
Sway your arm.
Turn your arm.
Let your arm fall to stand onto your shoulder blade, und so weiter ...

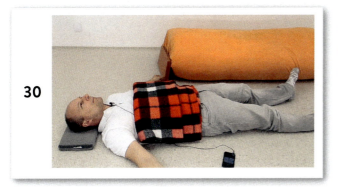

REST
Review this and the previous lessons in your mind. Rest.

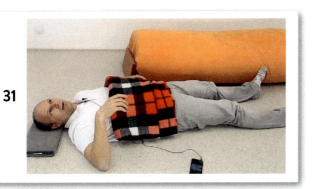

LET YOUR HAND SINK OVER
Try the first movement of this lesson again. Compare, how is it now?

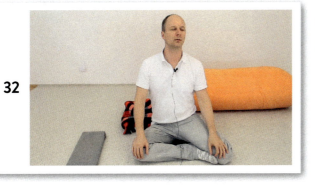

SIT UP
Float yourself into sitting. Feel yourself in sitting.

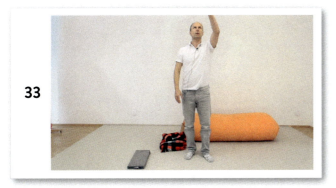

STAND UP
Float yourself up to standing. Use what you have learned in this lesson to come from sitting to standing. Don't hold your breath at any time, don't shorten your spine. Try lifting your arm in standing to see how it can float further up.

Jacqueline Remillard   1 year ago

Alfons, you rock! These lessons are AMAZING! They are helping me so much with my posture and neck pain. You are a wonderful teacher. I appreciate your kindness and generosity. I will share your channel with others. Thank you!

Dominique Deroiteau   11 months ago

superbe lesson... thanks ...the first time i didn t catch it too much ...this second time .... really my head up alone without effort ... and hips lights ! Merci !!!!

Mou Heaven   3 months ago

Thank you for sharing this lesson. I've play it over and over and find lots of joy while doing the movement. I have a quiestion: are the erector muscles the main muscles involved in the movements proposed in this lesson? Thank you for your help!! Congrats for such wonderful channel.

Maryline W   10 months ago

wonderful movements!
thank you a million times, Alfonso!

dominette   8 months ago

Awesome...again, the feeling in the body is amazing. The more I do, the more I feel and am beginning to understand Feldenkrais. I have to say that I have been able to do more without constantly hurting myself, whereas before I was constantly injuring my back..I an thrilled that I have been able to do things I haven't done in a long time because of only a few weeks following you and doing these classes.

Thank you so much

Olga Shmidov   1 year ago

Love love lessons could not believe what happened to my stiff neck   Is it possible to squeeze in 5 minutes for morning routine? Or is very important to be in slow pace? Thank you very much Alfons!!!! Looking forward for next video. Olga

Kevin Laing   11 months ago

Just got rid of my headache. These lessons are fab. Thankyou Alfons. I'm so grateful.

Penthesilea   2 months ago

You were pleasantly surprised when you lifted your head at the end and I was amazed too because my head floated up and brought my chest with me. My entire torso lifted up. Not exaggerating. These lessons are definitely not too slow. They are perfectly paced, for my needs anyway. I very much enjoy and appreciation your talking us through this, everything you say has meaning. Lastly, your exploration of the English language as we explore these lessons is so charming and fits perfectly with what we are trying to do.   Thank you, Alfons.

svetmes   11 months ago

The good lesson. It was interesting to explore lying on front. My back became soft like a butter). It's so great! Thank you.

Joshi Seeks   6 months ago

Dear Alfons, following your course here on youtube, this particular episode is absolutely stunning. Suffering from a serious chronicle spine related issue I just couldn´t do anything lying in prone for years. With this one session I could not only (not so easy though) follow it but felt rather well after practicing. Thank you for beeing so generous providing your knowledge.

Avery Joycelyn Barakuda Block   7 months ago

Well, I was just so put off by how slow and pokey you are and how long it takes you to krechts out a thought. And further irritated because in the back of my head -- back of my head - ha -- I'm disappointed with myself that I couldn't (didn't) slow down as I knew was appropriate.

But alas, I JUST KEPT WATCHING you in your little orange puffed blissfully empty room et voilà!: By the end of the second video I'm completely sold, completely engaged.

→Your absolutely exceptional expertise, so nuanced, so subtle is greatly appreciated.

All testimonial citations in this chapter are from publicly visible comments in the public comment section of my YouTube video „BETTER POSTURE WITHOUT STRETCHING OR WORKOUT?", https://goo.gl/gcsdKb, (December 6, 2017). I try to attribute as correctly as feasible, according to the official APA guidelines.

LESSON 6

Lifting your legs in prone position

During the first year of a child's life his mental growth is dependent on an unimpeded development of his motor abilities.

KAREL BOBATH AND BERTA BOBATH

PLEASE WORK THROUGH THE VIDEO FIRST TO BENEFIT FULLY FROM THIS *Workbook*

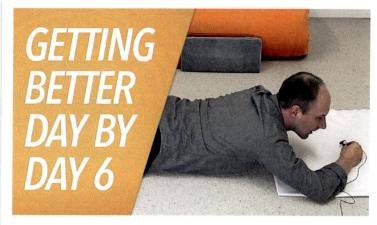

YOUTUBE VIDEO TITLE:
BETTER POSTURE WITHOUT STRETCHING OR WORKOUT?

Is there something like human growth and development? For sure we can say there's a lifelong process of physical, behavioural, cognitive, and emotional change. But then, is there? Do we change emotionally? Do we change how we move? There's charts and writings that tell what a human is likely to learn next – in terms of motor development, speech, vision, hearing, and social behaviour (and so forth) from pre-birth to birth, early childhood, toddlerhood, adolescence, adulthood all the way through seniority and death (stages of decay?). There's all sorts of systems that identify all sorts of stages of all sorts of development. What's the relevance of this? When do we need to refer to such a system? Which system do we pick? How valid is it for our purpose?

Maybe, for the sake of a lesson preface, it's easiest to say that there's people who gradually get better and people who gradually get worse… for example if we look at how people move. After big progress in their first years of life, for some people, little by little, and over the years, their movement repertoire is shrinking until they are unable to dress on their own or to take a shower without assistance. Maybe there's also people who gradually get worse at how they think, talk, feel, sense, interact. But is there the opposite too? Are there people who always keep improving? People who delight us with their acquired skills in certain fields? Or is it always a mix of all possibilities? What do psychologists have to say about this? What's in the basket of scholars, educators, researchers, religious leaders, authors, adventurers? What do the elderly have to report about this?

TUMMY TIME!

In this lesson we'll continue our journey through basic movement patterns. Specifically how to extend the spine, alas, the whole self, in lying prone. Tummy time! On one hand you'll be reviewing what you have (or should have) already learned as a toddler, on the other hand you're going to try a whole lot of new ideas and possibilities in quite a systematic way. One word of caution: take good care of your neck. If your neck hurts after only a few minutes in lying in a prone position (AKA on your belly) then turn your head around frequently or take frequent rests on your back.

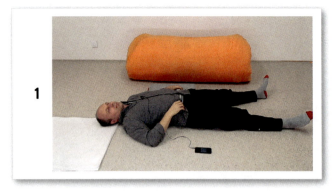

ARRIVE
Get on the floor and give yourself a minute or two. Take your time until your breathing is evenly and calm.

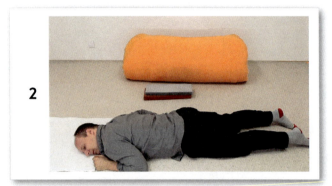

BREATHING IN PRONE POSITION
Feel how and where your breathing feels differently in prone position as opposed to supine position. The starting position for the next movements is in prone position, which means that the floor is now in front of you instead of behind of you.

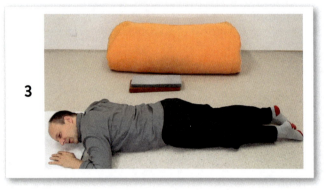

LIFT YOUR HEAD A TINY LITTLE BIT
Do merely an approximation, a first attempt in lifting your head, so small, that it should be almost unnoticeable from an outside perspective. In another video I called this „The postcard lift". Only lift your head high enough so that somebody could pull out a postcard that your resting on.

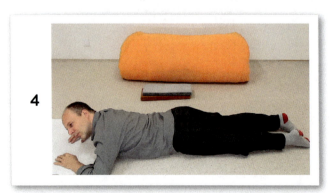

LIFT YOUR HEAD A LITTLE BIT MORE
Keep your hands somewhere next to your head. Explore the difference between pushing with your hands against the floor and lifting your head without the help of your arms.

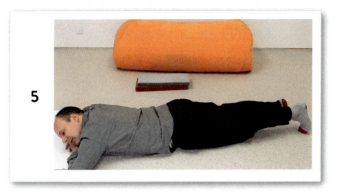

LIFT & EXTEND LEFT KNEE: POSITION 1

Place your hands on top of each other, with your head turned to the left. Stand the toes of your left foot next to your right foot (to the left of your right foot). Lift your left knee by extending (straightening) your left knee. You could think of pushing with your heel, push something away from you.

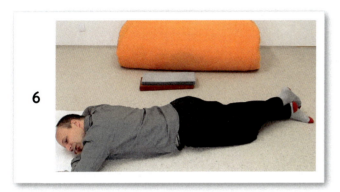

LIFT & EXTEND LEFT KNEE: POSITION 2

Place the instep of your left foot on the lower end of your calf muscles of your right leg, close to the heel of your right foot. In other words cross your left foot casually over your right leg, at the lower end of your right leg. Stand the toes of your left foot. Start to explore lifting your left knee again, keep the toes standing on the floor.

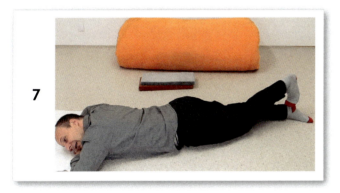

LIFT & EXTEND LEFT KNEE: POSITION 3

This time stand the toes of your left foot onto the heel of your right foot. A rather unusual position, isn't it? Start lifting your left knee again by extending your left leg.

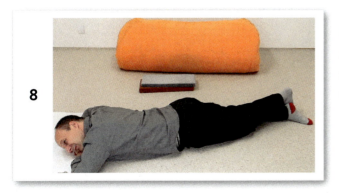

LIFT & EXTEND LEFT KNEE: POSITION 4

Stand your left foot crossed over your right leg, a bit further to the right of your right foot. Play a bit with various positions for your left foot.

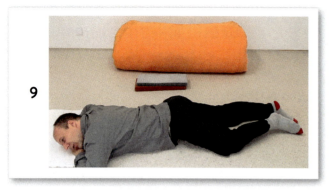

EXTEND AND FLEX YOUR KNEE

Continue these variations and explorations of lifting and extending the knee, but after letting your left knee sink to the floor bend your left knee a bit, just like in a crawling movement. Combine the flexion and extension of your knee into a smooth, continuous movement.

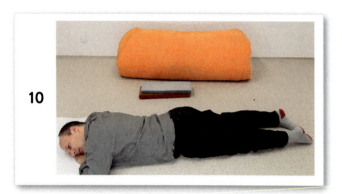

PAUSE

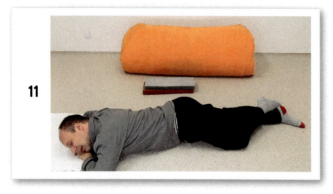

LIFT YOUR LEFT HIP JOINT

In prone position with your left leg a little bit bent (like in a crawling position) lift your left hip joint off the floor a tiny bit more. Increase the distance between your left anterior superior iliac spine and the floor, and then let yourself drop closer to the floor again. Let your left knee casually slide on the floor.

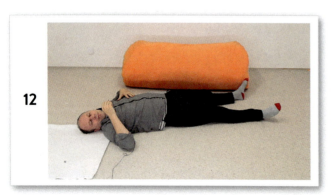

TAKE A BREAK ON YOUR BACK

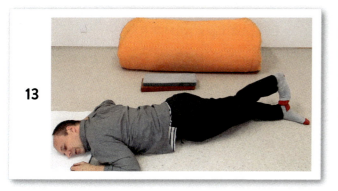

REVIEW
In prone position review the previous lifting and extension movements. See how it is now. Try again with the many different places where you can stand the toes of your left foot.

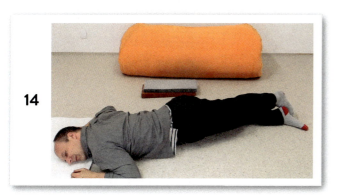

LIFT LEFT HIP JOINT AND LEFT KNEE
Now add the lifting of your left hip joint – the movement we just practiced [11]. Lift your left hip joint together with extending and lifting your left knee. Roll your pelvis back onto the floor when bending (flexing) your knee.

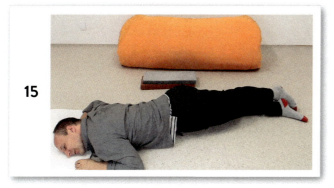

SEQUENCE LIFTING YOUR HIP JOINT AND EXTENDING YOUR KNEE
a) Lift hip joint first, then add extending and lifting your knee
b) Extend and lift knee first, then add lifting your hip joint
c) Lift both hip joint and knee together at the same time

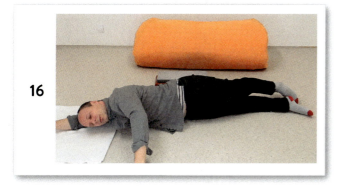

HELP WITH PUSHING HAND
Stand your left hand. Try different places and ways to stand your hand, then chose the one that makes the most sense. Continue the previous movement, but now add pushing with your left hand against the floor. Your whole torso will roll together with your pelvis. Place your right arm so that it allows this rolling movement to happen. Do whatever is necessary to make this smooth and comfortable.

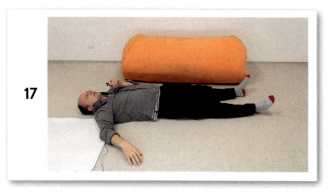

TAKE A BREAK ON YOUR BACK
Roll your head a bit to the left and right. Is there a difference between your left side and right side?

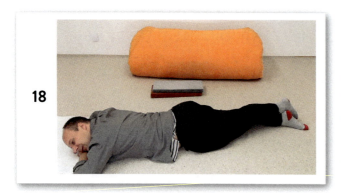

LIFT YOUR LEFT KNEE AGAIN
Back in prone position, place your left hand on top of right hand, your head on top of your left hand, your head turned to the left, your left knee bent like in crawling, your left foot crossed over your right leg. Return to the previous movements of lifting and extending your left knee. Has this movement improved? What's different in your sensing and feeling?

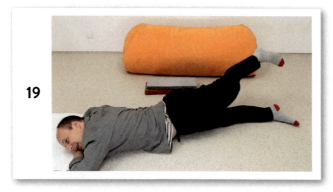

LIFT YOUR LEFT LEG UP HIGHER
Continue the movement of extending and lifting your left knee to lifting your entire left leg. Involve your pelvis, your whole self. You might want to think of dancing Tango. However, don't let your elbows or head leave the floor.

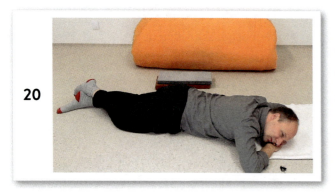

REPEAT THE ENTIRE SEQUENCE ON THE OTHER SIDE
This time lift and bend your right knee, do all the movements we just did, but on the other side.

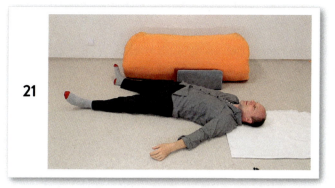

REST
Take a rest on your back and compare how it is to the beginning of the lesson.

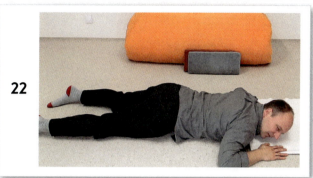

LIFT BOTH HIP JOINTS AT THE SAME TIME
Back to prone position. Instead of lifting just one hip joint, rise both hip joints away from the floor at the same time. It looks a little bit like humping the floor in slow motion. Technically it's an extension of your back initiated from your hip joint (instead of lifting your head, which would mean initiating the extension of your spine from your head). Lift your hip joints and the let your pelvis drop to the floor again.

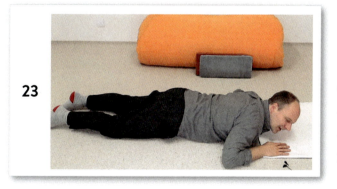

LIFT YOUR HEAD
Now, there we have the extension of the spine starting with your head (is it?). Compare to the beginning of this lesson. Sense the connection through your whole spine, chest, to your pelvis, down to your knees and feet. At which areas do you lean against the floor?

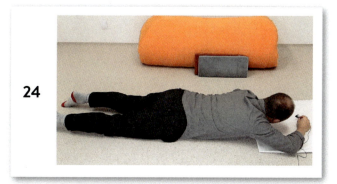

LIFT YOUR HEAD IN VARIATIONS
Lift, rest, lift and turn your head, rest in various places. Don't stop your breathing while lifting.

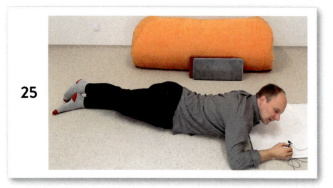

LIFT YOUR LEG AND HEAD

Still in prone position lift one hip joint and/or one knee while lifting the head. Put it all together, involve your whole self. Play, enjoy.

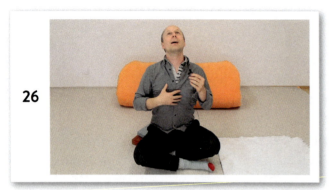

SIT UP

Feel how it is in sitting. Play a bit with extending the head (looking up) in sitting.

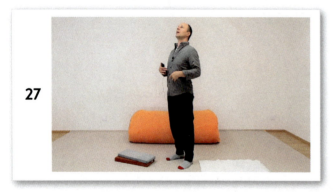

STAND UP

See how it is in standing.

♥ Jane McLaren 1 year ago

Thanks always. After doing this lesson my ability to feel myself breathing into my back became very easy and strangely pleasant. My neck became very free, too. Looking forward to the next lesson.

J Algar 1 year ago

Thank you, Alfons. I noticed a big difference in the way my neck had more freedom of movement. As always, I look very forward to the next video. You are so appreciated!

Adrian Katzenstein 11 months ago

Room room room! lol man this is great i always thought i needed something not as complex as most videos that always makes my neck hurt more or gives me headaches, i love your method easy to follow and easy on the body! appreciate these

Phil Gardner 1 year ago

Thanks for this lesson...yes, really noticed the head and neck floating over the shoulders and much more openness in the chest. My shoulders felt much more back (less rounded) without effort.

Raphaëlle Nime 8 months ago

3.333 views! Now go for 33.333, you deserve it :-)
Thank you so much.

♥

allonespirit1 — 1 month ago

I have been following this series now for a week. I am not able to do all the movements you do but I do what I can a few times and then watch the rest of the video and imagine doing it. I have been chronically ill for over ten years and cannot walk more than half a block.

Today I went to my chiropractor for the first time in 2 months. She confirmed that my chest has become unlocked, my breathing deeper, my left shoulder can now lie flat on the bed for the first time in 25 yrs! She was amazed at the changes and my body awareness. I wanted to pass this on to you. I do one or maybe 2 exercises a day.

I love your teaching style and the way you make the lessons easily broken down. You are a wonderful teacher and awareness coach. 🌹🌹🧡

Julie Fitzgerald — 1 year ago

I enjoyed this lesson. The best part of all was the invitation to explore and find my own easiest way to do these movements. Honoring the integrity of one's body while incorporating new discoveries, is as you say, "a practice of self respect and love". Thank you!

Maud v — 1 year ago

I had a shoulder o.p bankart, 3 months ago, in this lesson I started with my arm 45 degrees next to my body. Your starting position was impossible for me. But by the end of the lesson, I could put my arm in the starting position. Whoohooo. Thats a big thing. Thanx

Following My Bliss — 1 year ago

I feel myself there fore I am. That's profound. I never "THOUGHT" about Descarte's statement 'I THINK I am since I heard it in my early teens. How ironic...

Lucy Choisser — 1 year ago

The lessons and your teaching this series (and other lessons too!) have been very helpful in pain relief, ease in movement, alignment, and posture improvement. Thank you so much!

Adrian Katzenstein — 10 months ago

I just did lesson 6 and 7 right now and felt awesome, the first day i started my head felt like a bowling ball, now it is starting to feel lighter and can turn easier! not to mention more relaxed and aware.

AliveandReconnected — 8 months ago

I was surprised to notice that after the first time doing this lesson my long-standing (over 60 years) reverse curve in my neck has gone and is replaced with a normal curve! I have been using a soft woolen neck roll to sleep on, and have done so for years, but this is the first time I have a normal curve in my cervical spine. I just repeated this lesson and notice this time how 'right' my chest and lungs feel: both spacious and relaxed....thanks, Alfons

Donni Hakanson — 1 year ago

Thankyou Alfons, I am a fan! You are a very engaging teacher with humor, I enjoy your lessons and the differences I feel in my body. I first knew of Feldenkrais half a life time ago and have a few books by Moshe and others, but didn't get to attend my first lessons until two years ago. I like being able to follow along at home and be able to see what you are doing if I'm not sure. Thankyou again, it's wonderful you are sharing these series of classes!

Allen Adamson — 1 year ago

I've been practising Feldenkrais movements for six months or more, using your YouTube videos. These last two lessons have been the most difficult but satisfying. I was very aware of tension in the opposite side in the gluteus (buttocks) as I was lifting the head and elbow I.e. Lifting the right elbow produced tension in the left gluteus.

Silja Sjödin — 1 year ago

really deep relaxing just watching your video, being totally focused on the instructions and the movements, like being aware 100% in body presence....this was my third video Feldenkrais with Alfons, first time I've ever heard about Feldenkrais was yesterday when doing research on injured foot rehab and I stoped for watching a ballerina having some F- theraphy to heal her foot... very, very, very interesting to listen to you Alfons, no I don't think the video is too long...maybe the lingering in instruction and repetition of description creates the perfect slow down mood to understand with the body how it should be done in the right way. Thanks

All testimonial citations in this chapter are from publicly visible comments in the public comment section of my YouTube video „WHAT IS TRAUMA? HOW TO RESOLVE IT?", https://goo.gl/Wyyvms, (December 7, 2017). I try to attribute as correctly as feasible, according to the official APA guidelines.

LESSON 7

Lifting your head in prone position

For my patients I always recommend that they see somebody who helps them to really feel their body, experience their body, open up to their bodies.

BESSEL VAN DER KOLK

PLEASE WORK THROUGH THE
VIDEO FIRST
TO BENEFIT FULLY FROM THIS
Workbook

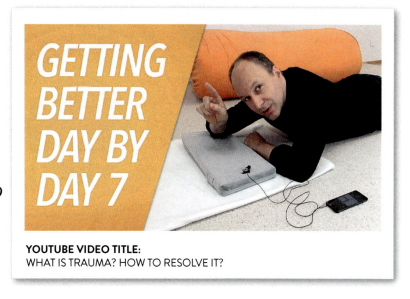

YOUTUBE VIDEO TITLE:
WHAT IS TRAUMA? HOW TO RESOLVE IT?

In this lesson we'll pick up the theme from the previous lesson (extension) and build on it. You will explore how arm movements, breathing, and eye movements affect and improve extension of your spine, alas, of your entire self.

ORGANIC

FELDENKRAIS® lessons certainly are not a „cure all". In fact FELDENKRAIS® is not even therapy, and FELDENKRAIS® practitioners are not therapists, at least not where I come from – Austria/Europe. I wouldn't call ourselves movement teachers either. As FELDENKRAIS® Practitioners we try to provide an environment (a setting?) for learning. We do this through talking and touching. For human beings learning, and especially organic learning, is a biological, not to say physiological, necessity. „Trauma" is said to be a big umbrella term that includes physical and emotional events (and probably much more). It's a big topic, to say the least. To quote Dr. Moshé Feldenkrais: „You can see that one real trauma, real painful trauma, lasts for some people a lifetime. They need afterwards to be ten or fifteen years in psychotherapy to get rid of it and maybe can't; they don't get rid of it anyway because it's impossible to limit. It's connected to so many different... associated with so many different things, that suddenly you think you're fine and a real good association brings it back." In his book „The Elusive Obvious" he writes: „How many practice Zen, meditation, psychoanalysis by several different methods, psychodrama, biofeedback, hypnotism, dance therapy, and so on. There must be something like fifty or more known therapies for people who do not feel medically ill, but are discontented with their sensations and performance. In all the methods we have to help people in distress they do a considerable amount of learning. So we have to understand the different kinds of learning before we can see the importance of yet another method created and used by me."

EXTENSION

FELDENKRAIS® lessons help us to get out of our heads and into our bodies. They help us to improve how we interact with the world. Is that true? How does this work?

FELDENKRAIS® lessons give us the opportunity to bond with ourselves, to make peace not only with gravity, but with reality, and to be able to act in this world without feeling burdened by our inabilities.

Let's see how this lesson flows with the topic. Maybe let's start with lying on the floor, take a good rest, and then let's start with these extension movements. Extension. Expansion. Gracefully growing towards our full potential again…

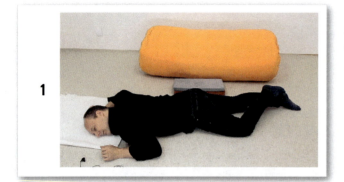

ARRIVE
Take a few moments to arrive at the floor, we will start in prone position.

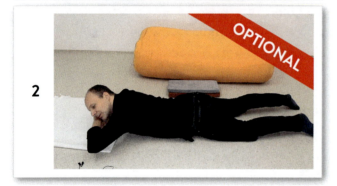

LIFT YOUR HEAD TOGETHER WITH YOUR HAND AND ELBOW
In prone position, with your head turned to the left, your head on top of your left hand, your left hand on top of your right hand, try this „reference movement". It's like a test, and we will do this again at the end of the lesson and compare how it changed. How easy or hard is it? What do you notice?

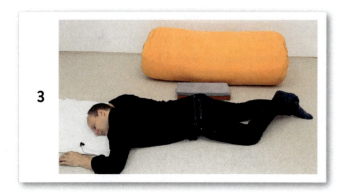

SLIDE HAND UPWARDS
Rest again, in prone position, with your head turned to the left. As a first movement slide your left hand upwards, away from your head. Then drag it back downwards somewhere to its starting position. Do this in a very relaxed fashion. Feel how your elbow pushes and pulls your hand. If it feels more comfortable, safer, or more natural to do, you can also start with dragging your hand downwards first (why is this different?).

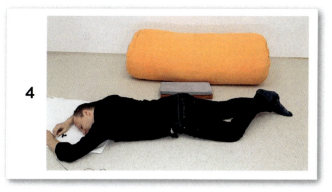

SLIDE HAND UPWARDS TOWARDS YOUR MIDLINE

As before, slide your hand up and above your head, but this time steer towards an imaginary midline, not just upwards or going to the left.

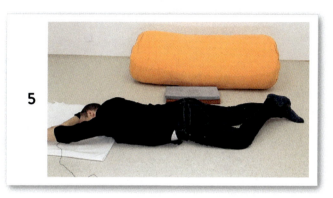

SLIDE YOUR HAND AND LIFT YOUR ELBOW

While sliding your elbow upwards, also lift your elbow off the floor. Find the right moment to do so. It's a similar movement as in the last lesson, only now it's about lifting and extending your arm instead of your leg.

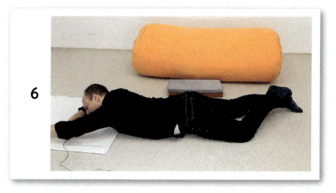

SLIDE YOUR HAND THEN LIFT YOUR ELBOW AND YOUR HAND

In addition to your elbow also lift your hand off the floor. In this way, gradually, lift your entire arm off the floor … If you like think of your hand holding a toy aeroplane taking off.

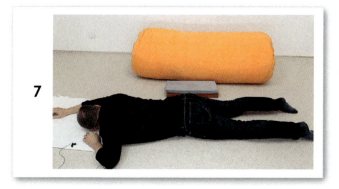

SAME WITH YOUR RIGHT ARM

Turn your face to the right. Work through the same lifting sequence [3-6] with your right arm.

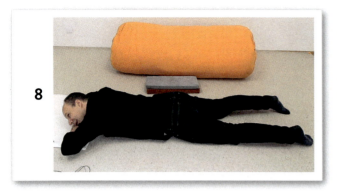

LIFT YOUR HEAD, HAND AND ELBOW SIMULTANEOUSLY

In prone position, with your head turned to the left, your right ear on the back of your left hand, your left hand on top of your right hand. Start lifting in following order:

1. lift your LEFT elbow a little bit
2. lift your head a little bit
3. lift your left hand and head together
4. lift your hand, head and elbow together, slowly.

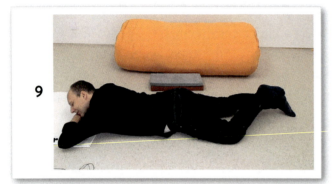

LIFT AGAIN, BUT IN A CURVED PATHWAY

Lift your arm+hand+head concoction again, but this time do it by sliding your elbow upwards first, on a curved pathway rather than straight lifting. Allow yourself to lengthen.

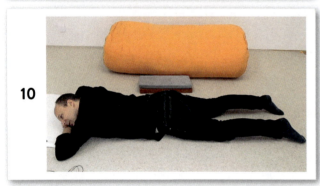

LIFT YOUR RIGHT HAND AND ELBOW

Your head still turned to the left, resting on top of your right hand, your right hand on top of your left hand. Start lifting in the following order:

1. lift your right elbow
2. lift your head
3. lift your head and RIGHT hand
4. lift all together, allow yourself to rise on a curved pathway

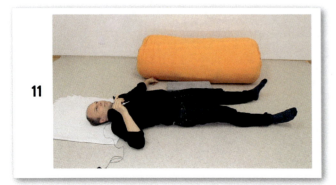

REST ON YOUR BACK

Take a short rest on your back. Feel how you are resting on the floor, feel your shoulder blades, spine, buttocks etc

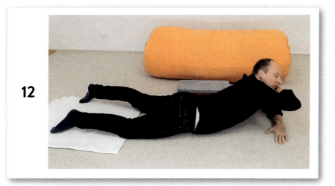

REPEAT ON THE OTHER SIDE
Play through the same sequence [7-10], but with your head turned to the right, lifting your right arm and head together. Don't rush through it, take your time (what is that, „your time"?)

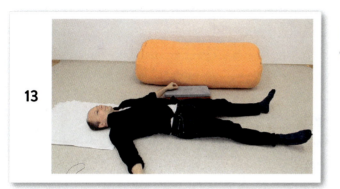

REST ON YOUR BACK
Take a break in supine position and see how it is.

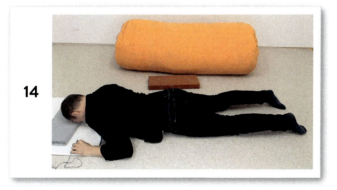

**LOOK DOWNWARDS,
WITH YOUR EYES ONLY**
In prone position, with your forehead resting on your hands or a cushion, your head not turned sideways but facing forwards (to the floor). Just with your eyes: gradually look downwards, towards your feet.

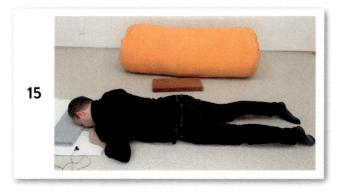

**LOOK UPWARDS,
WITH YOUR EYES ONLY**
Just with your eyes: gradually look upwards, the direction is towards your hairline. Don't lift your head, don't move anything else (too much).

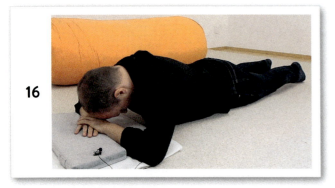

LOOK DOWNWARDS
Look downwards towards your feet, but this time also involve your neck and shoulders and eyes.

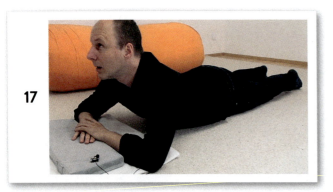

LOOK UPWARDS
Look upwards and lift your head, involve your eyes, your neck, your shoulders, lean against your chest. Feel how to point of contact with the floor travels, feel with which area of yourself you lean against the floor in each moment.

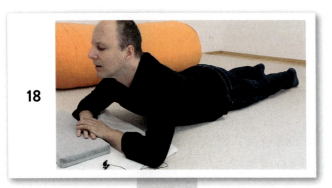

EYE MOVEMENTS IN OPPOSITE DIRECTION OF HEAD MOVEMENTS
Lift your head while you look downwards with your eyes, do these two things at the same time, well coordinated. It might be quite difficult at first.

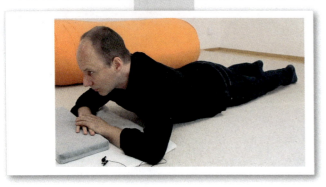

Then look upwards (with your eyes) and at the same time lower your head. You might need a couple of attempts and some time to get used to this. Do this gradually, don't panic.

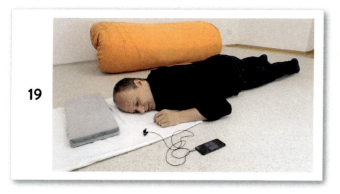

TAKE A REST
Much earned.

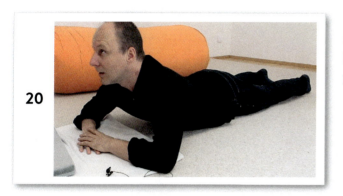

REVIEW: LIFT YOUR HEAD AND LOOK UP SIMULTANEOUSLY
Look up and lift your head. How is it now?

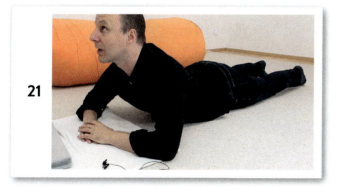

ADD BREATHING TO LIFTING
While you breath in lift your head and eyes. Coordinate everything together to move smoothly and attentively. Feel how and where you lean against the floor with your chest.

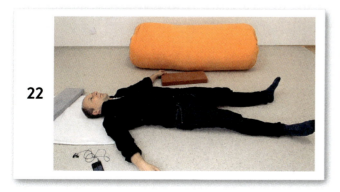

TAKE A BREAK ON YOUR BACK
How do you breath now? How and where do you feel your chest now?

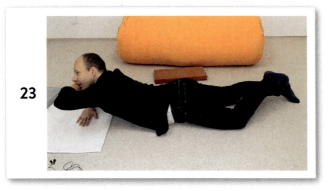

LIFT YOUR HEAD TOGETHER WITH YOUR HAND AND ELBOW

Get into prone position with your head turned to the left, your right ear on the back of your left hand, your left hand on top of your right hand. Lift your head and left arm together. This is the reference movement from the beginning of this lesson. See how it has changed. How is it now?

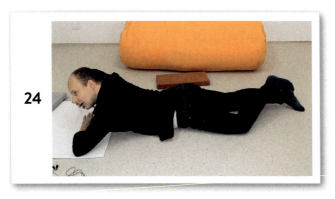

LIFT YOUR HEAD TOGETHER WITH YOUR RIGHT HAND AND ELBOW

Try this variation too: in prone position, your head still turned to the left, your right ear on the back of your right hand, your right hand on top of your left hand. Lift your head and right arm together.

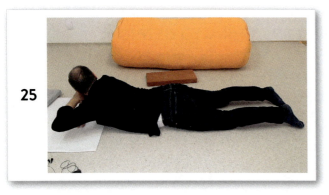

ON THE OTHER SIDE

Also try these same two lifting variations with your head turned to the right.

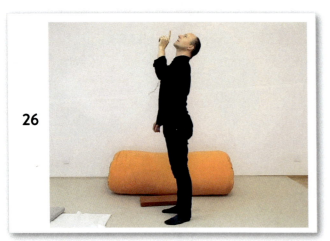

SIT UP AND STAND UP

Feel how it is in standing

Emily Eyre 5 months ago

i can't lie down on my front side without pain...it hurts when my chest is pressing against the floor. does this mean i should avoid doing any movements that require me to lay face down?

Emily Eyre 4 months ago

thank you! i really enjoyed doing the last five lessons again since it truly is a new experience each time! after repeating the previous lessons i came back to this one and suddenly no longer found it painful to lay on my front side! thank you for your advice and i look forward to exploring more body movements!

AliveandReconnected 8 months ago

Alfons, it is always a treat to follow your lessons! I have experienced repeated whiplash, thoracic spine and neck trauma in early childhood, as well as sexual abuse. Injuries as an adult, as well. I was a little stiff and uncomfortable in the beginning of this lesson. My increased mobility and ease at the end of the lesson were wonderful- and interestingly enough, my shoulders feel light, broader and spacious- for the first time! My eyes feel soft, heavy and relaxed, so I'm finding this lesson's effects are both widespread and potent. My whole upper body has loosened and my chest feels lifted (more room for air!) I'm also pleased that your book arrived today from Amazon! :-)
Many thanks!

John Moseley 8 months ago

I was interested in this lesson for addressing emotional trauma, but, ironically, of all the lessons I've done of yours, this was the one that ended up helping me most with physical pain. About a month ago, I fell over on some slippery tiles and twisted my right shoulder. I didn't think it was actually injured and never saw a doctor about it, but it's been very sore ever since and a lot less flexible. Flexibility hasn't completely returned, but the pain, amazingly, in ordinary positions, seems to be gone. Maybe it was partly something to do with the fact that this was a lesson that felt like it could have made it worse, but, in line with your teaching, I was always trying to do it in a way that wouldn't hurt. Thanks, Alfons! Feldenkrais is a revelation and your brilliant lessons are something I've quickly come to value very much.

Phil Gardner 1 year ago

I liked this lesson, like the rest, but I didn't notice so much improvement in the head lifting. I could lift the arm and head fairly easily at the beginning and end. The big improvement was in how my head sat back on the shoulders when standing, and how much more open the chest is. I have had a couple of bad injuries in my neck - one when I fell on my head on a trampoline and it bent to one side with all my body weight on top....so I noticed that when doing the exercise where we would lie with the forehead on the floor and look up and down, whenever I looked down there is pain in the vertebrae in my neck. I am really interested in these lessons to help with this sort of old injury, but much more interested in the resolving of old trauma - I have been working on this from both a mental and emotional perspective for many years, using meditation and inquiry techniques - so this is fascinating using a physical method. Thank you.

Bruno Varela 11 months ago

Hello Alfons! Many thank yous for your youtube channel and for sharing your Feldenkrais knowledge with us. This lesson was just great for me today. I had a busy day and some pain in my low back, but after the lesson I felt wonderful. Your lessons are very good and I enjoy them a lot.

Raphaëlle Nime 8 months ago

Thank you for this lesson... I happened to SING after it and got very much surprised: the voice was much more open, flexibel, strong and articulated! I recommend this way of freeing the neck for every singer! Genial.

Johan Roy D'souza 1 year ago

Alright so here it is my actual comment on My Seventh Day!!! I have been having a stiff neck and weak upper back muscles for the past 8 months and been doing physio to recover. I feel great on my Seventh Day. I have been doing this method alongside my physio exercises but I must say that I get a great feeling after the Feldenkrais sessions more than the strengthning exercises. Unfortunately there are no Feldenkrais teachers where I live so this channel is a gift. Thanks a lot Alfons.

Mariana Letelier 3 weeks ago

I ended the lesson saying "weeeeeeeeeeeeeeee"... heheheh... i am really enjoying the series. Thank you very much!! My body had gone through so many changes that i am not sure how it is suposed to be anymore. I'll do all your lessons. Thanks a lot again.

Leah Twitchell 1 year ago

I felt so fluid at the end of this lesson... like a jellyfish. This was definitely the funnest so far!! ;) Also, that onesie is ah-mazing. I need one of those. I would wear it all winter.

annandmore 1 year ago

I nearly felt out of my bed :)). really proper funny, thx.

Avery Joycelyn Barakuda Block 7 months ago

The fact is, for some of us this Must be difficult. Certainly not comfortable. My plan to get around this, because I do intend to get to comfort or some kind of ease, is to Feel my discomfort as something that I am traveling Through rather than an immovable fate. I'm trying to keep organic sensibility while lifting all these different parts here into the 35 min. point I got the idea to see myself -- FEEL myself -- as deep down in the very colorful oceanic realm. Even better ~ to be an octopus. Big difference toward conceptualising the gesture(s). I'm going to go with Quadropus, though the head should probably be included.

Ein besonderer Youtubeuser 2 weeks ago

For me it was a little bit too much. Maybe i have to use the pause-Button. I will repeat it. But thank you for so much Input and i felt great after it. Really love that rolling

Anth8787 7 months ago

Alfons, this listen is such a great experience after doing the previous seven lessons. Feeling my ability to roll over, initiating with my legs, and then later with arms, is a very empowering feeling. Thank you so much!!

Deena Spaner 4 months ago

Hi alfonse! First, thank you for sharing! It was difficult to find any feldenkrais lessons lead by a real person on YouTube. I've been following you getting better day by day even though I have some feldenkrais experience already I'm really enjoying it..

Raphaëlle Nime 8 months ago

AMAZING :-)

lenny3210 6 months ago

This is healing!

Yogi Bee 11 months ago

Thank you sooooo much for making these videos. They are excellent, you're a marvellous teacher. And thanks for the laughs too!

Lorry Onosson 2 months ago

Ahh, you like Peter Draws too! That is great! You are re-inspiring me, to feel better, and maybe to draw again! Thanks!

Penthesilea 2 months ago

Just finished 7 & 8. Didn't comment on 7 because I wanted to flow into 8 right away. Lovely feelings, thank you.

Myriam Russer 1 year ago

chest is inspired by movements of neck....its more than doodeling, right! :)

Rashid Elnoor 1 year ago

I feel good rest in my body thanks for the video happy times

All testimonial citations in this chapter are from publicly visible comments in the public comment section of my YouTube video „ROLLING ON THE FLOOR LIKE MOVEMENT PROS", https://goo.gl/pW8hvW, (December 9, 2017). I try to attribute as correctly as feasible, according to the official APA guidelines.

LESSON 8

Rolling over easily using everything you've got

The limits of my language are the limits of my world.

LUDWIG WITTGENSTEIN

PLEASE WORK THROUGH THE
VIDEO FIRST
TO BENEFIT FULLY FROM THIS
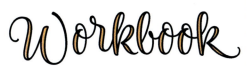

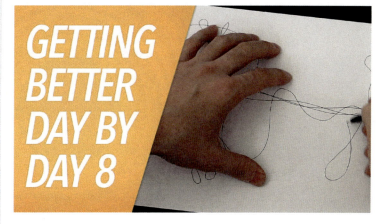

YOUTUBE VIDEO TITLE:
ROLLING ON THE FLOOR LIKE MOVEMENT PROS

When people think about movement they often think in straight lines. Left – right. Up – down. Forwards – backwards. Movement professionals usually use a more sophisticated vocabulary, e. g. physical therapists might use words like flexion, extension, translation, and rotation in anatomical planes called sagittal, horizontal and frontal.

However, I guess most people do not think in terms of movement at all. We simply don't have to. We don't have to study neuroscience and the mathematics of proprioception to be able to do stuff. Our nervous system does it all for us. Not out of the box certainly, but any half decent developed human being merely needs to focus on the tasks at hand to be able to successfully move through space. All the movement related stuff will somehow magically happen on its own. We don't need to think about how to lift an arm or how to turn the head.

OPPORTUNITY

In his book „The Elusive Obvious" Dr. Moshé Feldenkrais writes: „As it turns out, socially successful, very clever, important, creative people may devote no time to their personal growth. They find their whole life is their work, ignoring themselves far too often. Such people listen to me seriously only when they are incapacitated one way or another. Even so, I have reached by now thousands of them through their misfortunes." What kind of events, misfortunes, lucky coincidences, inspirations or opportunities make us listen? Or could we just listen, voluntarily?

For the upcoming lesson I want you to be inspired by the freedom of movement that is available to you, the many complex pathways you can move through, discover, explore, feel, sense, think about. I invite you to enter a world of movement that lies beyond any simple vocabulary or explanations. And even though the suggested movement opportunities might not look like much to a spectator, for the committed student they are nothing short of spectacular.

Discovering and following your own lines of movement, the lines of movement of your own choosing, can be a form of art, an expression of who you are and an expansion of your world. Moreover, it can be a beautiful way of accomplishing a meaningful task: to roll over from your back onto your belly, and back again.

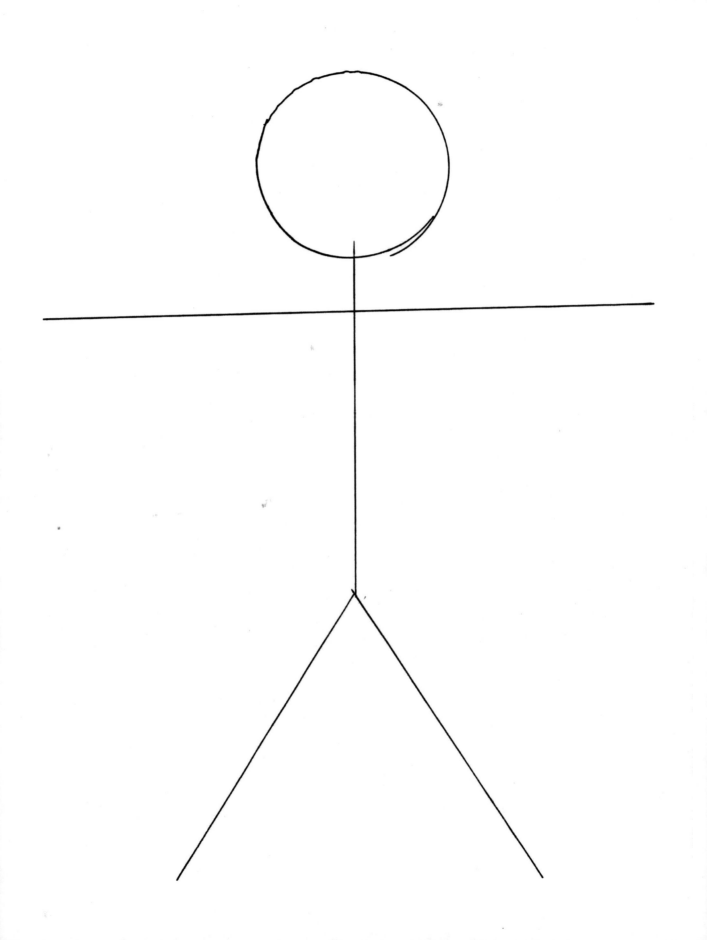

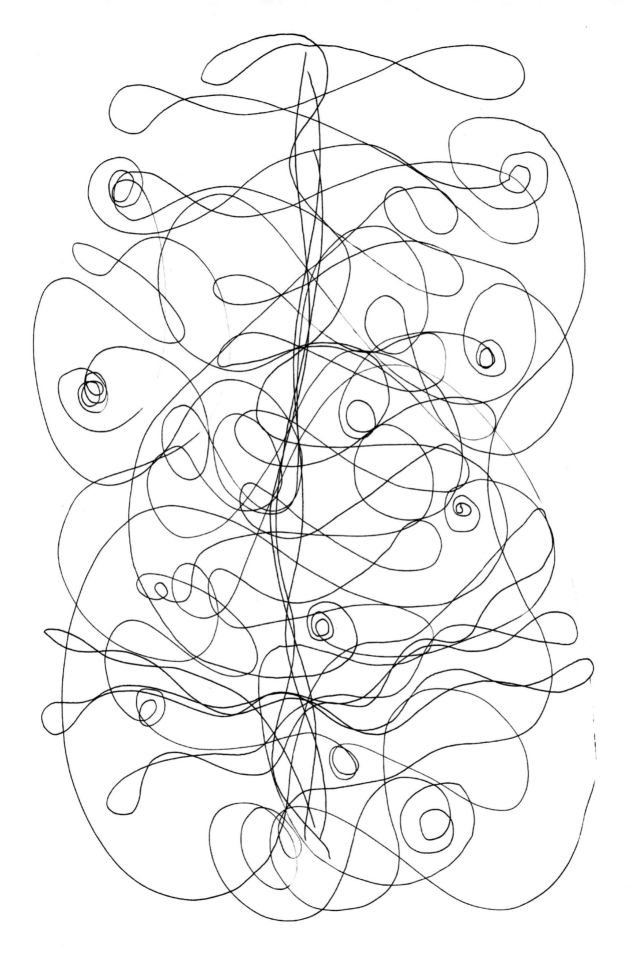

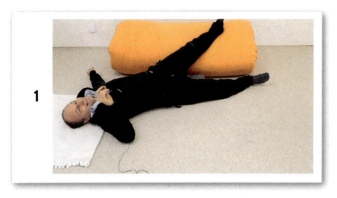

ARRIVE ON THE FLOOR

Before we start come to lie in a supine position on the floor. How long does it take to relax to the floor? 1 second, 10 seconds, 1 minute, 10 minutes? Maybe it's different every time? How do you know that you're relaxed and ready?

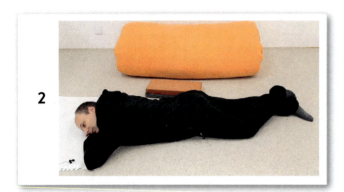

GET INTO THE STARTING POSITION

Prone position, your head turned to the left, your left hand on top of your right hand, your left foot hooked over the lower end of your right leg.

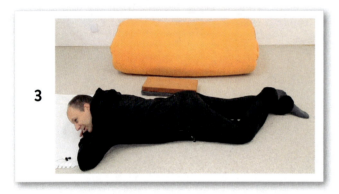

LIFT YOUR HEAD

Lift your head a tiny little bit and let it sink back down again. Think of the many things you have learned so far in the previous lessons about how you can lift your head.

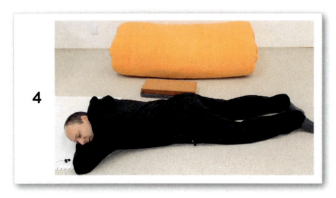

REST YOUR HEAD IN VARIOUS POSITIONS (FORWARDS)

Lift your head and then rest your head in a position a tiny bit more forwards, closer to your left elbow. Lift again, rest again. Repeat. Once you reached your elbow work your way back to the center again.

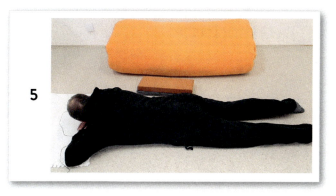

REPEAT WITH HEAD TO THE RIGHT

Place your right hand on top of your left hand, with your head turned to the right. Do the same explorations as before [3-4]. Notice if your chest is touching the floor stronger with your left side of your chest than it did before when you were facing to the left.

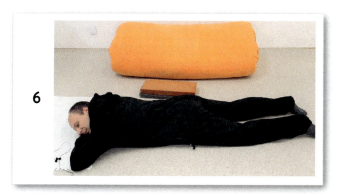

TAKE A REST

Take good care of your neck, turn it to the other side or turn or move your head frequently to avoid neck pain.

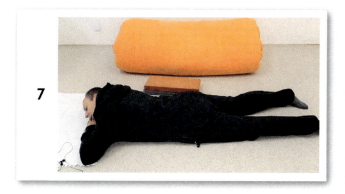

REST YOUR HEAD IN VARIOUS POSITIONS (BACKWARDS)

Have your head turned to the left (face to the left). Keep your head turned to the left. Lift your head and then place your head in a new position, closer to your right elbow. This means you're moving your head backwards. Think of the back of your head going backwards. Do not turn your head.

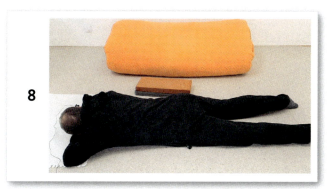

SAME ON THE OTHER SIDE

Repeat the same exploration [7] with your head turned to the right (face to the right). With every little lift bring your head closer to your left elbow. Do not turn your head, keep facing to the right. You may move everything except your elbows. Your elbows have to stay on the floor, your hands have to stay on top of each other.

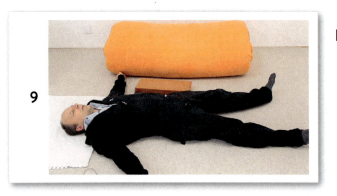

REST ON YOUR BACK

9

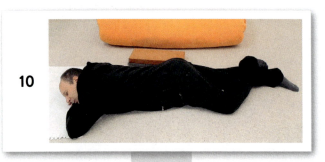

REVIEW LEG EXTENSION MOVEMENTS

Briefly review the leg movements from LESSON 6. Make them fluid and match them together. These are crawling-like movements.

10

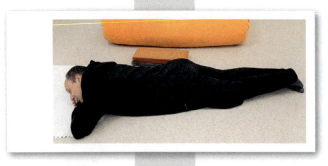

Straightening the left knee and lift your leg in various positions and pathways.

Straight..

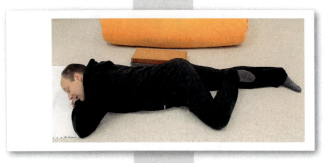

and bent...

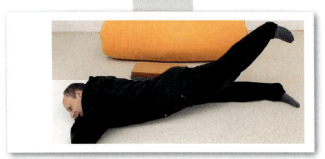

As a last movement lift your left leg higher, over your midline, over your right leg. Also try to extend it far out to the left, then find what is most easy. You could say it's a bit of a dance move, but while lying on your belly.

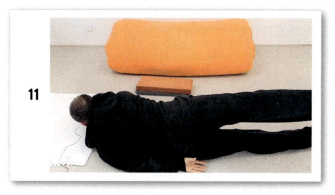

REVIEW LEG EXTENSION MOVEMENTS, ON THE OTHER SIDE

Briefly review the same explorations as just now, but on the other side, with your head turned to the right.

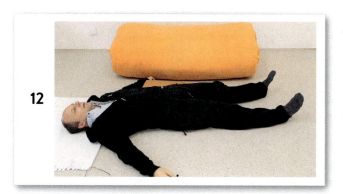

TAKE A SHORT BREAK

Preferably on your back.

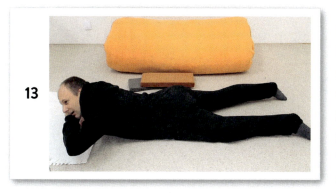

LIFT YOUR LEFT ARM AND YOUR HEAD, ON CURVED PATHWAYS

Start from prone position, with your left hand on top of your right hand, your head turned to the left, and your legs in any position you like. Lift your left arm and head together in curved pathways (not straight up and down, but following the natural lines of movement). Bring them down to rest in the same position as you started of.

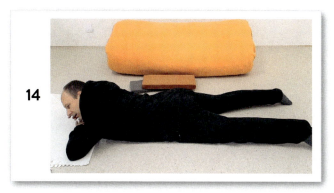

LIFT RIGHT ARM AND HEAD

With your head still turned to the left, but with your right hand on top of your left hand, lift your right arm and head together in curved pathways. Again bring them down to rest in the same position as you started.

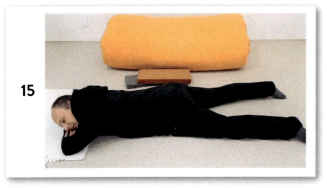

LIFT RIGHT ARM AND HEAD, REST IN VARIOUS POSITIONS

Starting position is with your head turned to the left, resting it on the back of your right hand (just like before). Lift your right hand + right elbow + head together. After every time you lifted your right hand (together with your right elbow and head) bring them down to a different position and fully rest for a couple of seconds (or doze off, any length of rest is allowed). Also try to rest in a position where your right hand (and head) is close to your left elbow.

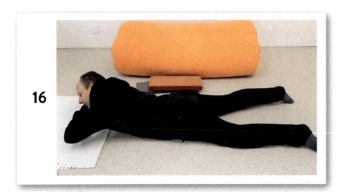

LIFT LEFT ARM AND HEAD, REST IN VARIOUS POSITIONS

This time have your head turned to the left and resting on your left hand. Your left hand resting on your right hand. Lift your left hand and head and entire left arm and then rest your head in various different positions.

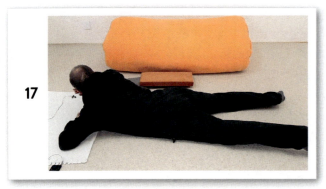

REPEAT ON THE OTHER SIDE

Explore the same four movements as before, but with your head turned to the right. Indeed [13-16] are four different variations.

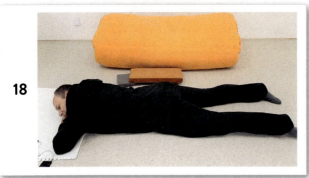

TAKE A SHORT REST

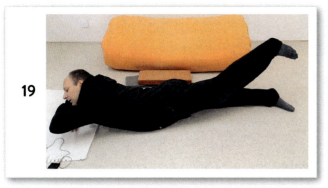

LIFT LEFT ARM AND LEFT LEG

Use everything you've learned so far. Lengthen. Be at ease. Float. Curve. Make your left side (and yourself) shorter (on the floor) and longer (in the air). Move slowly. Never strain yourself. Make frequent pauses.

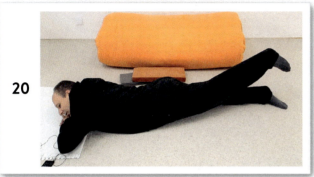

SLOW ROCKING MOTION

Whenever you rise your arm and head, lower your leg. Whenever you rise your leg, lower your arm and head. When you think of „your arm" do you think of your elbow? Your forearm? Your shoulder? Feel how and where the point of contact with the floor travels up and down on your front side.

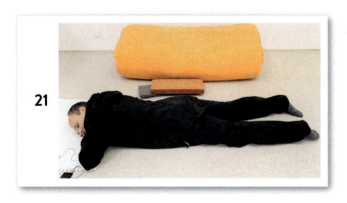

TAKE A BREAK

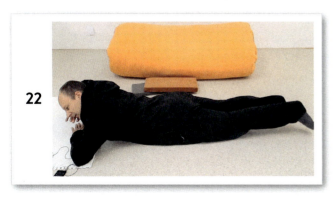

DIAGONAL LIFTING

With your head turned to the left, rest your head on top of your right hand, your right hand on top of your left hand. Lift your head together with your right arm. Lift your left leg. Lift them at the same time. Lift them in slow motion. Feel the point of contact on the floor. Where is it? At your pubic bone, navel, chest? Compare how this is different to before, when you did same side lifting and rocking [20].

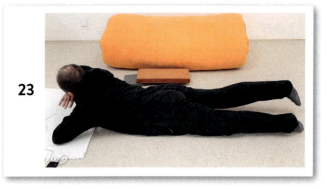

REPEAT LIFTING AND ROCKING ON THE OTHER SIDE

With your head turned to the right, lift your right arm and right leg, then your right arm and left leg. Find good, pleasant ways to do this. Do progress in approximations, do experiments, rest frequently and review.

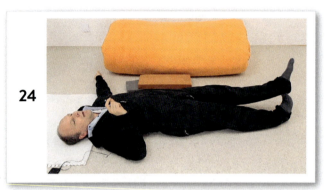

TAKE A PROPER REST ON YOUR BACK

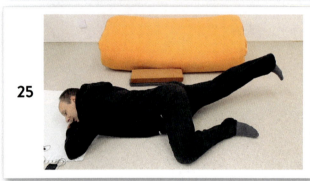

WITH YOUR LEFT LEG BENT, LIFT YOUR RIGHT LEG

In prone position again, get into following starting position: your head turned to the left, rest your head on top of your left hand, your left hand on top of your right hand, **your left leg pulled up into a crawling position**, and your right leg extended. Start by straightening your right knee, lift your right knee off the floor. Then add more and more until you can lift of your right leg. Experiment, review, explore. What difference does the bent left leg make?

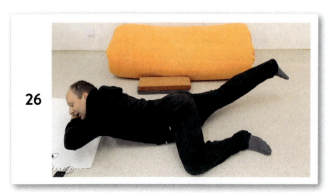

AGAIN WITH YOUR LEFT LEG BENT, LIFT YOUR LEFT ARM AND RIGHT LEG

Again with your left leg bent, start with lifting your left arm and head, re-examine the various pathways, play, explore. Then add lifting your right leg.

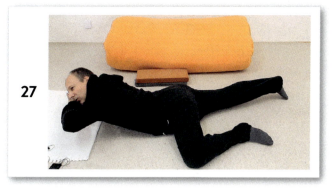

ROCKING MOTION FROM LEFT ELBOW TO RIGHT FOOT

You left leg still in a crawling position. Whenever you lift your left arm and head, lower your right leg. When you lower your left arm and head, lift your right leg. Find the connection. You can elongate your left arm if you like. Think, move, sense, feel.

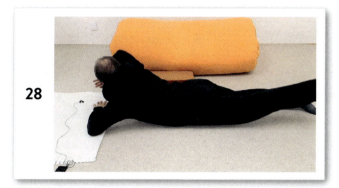

SAME ON THE OTHER SIDE

This time have your right leg bent. With this starting position, go through the previous variations:

1. lift your left leg,
2. then lift your right arm and head,
3. then your arm and head and leg at the same time
4. at last find the rocking motion

Lift, rock, pivot, make it big.

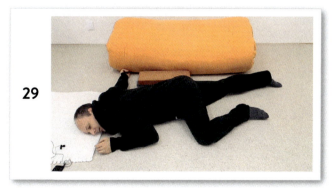

TAKE A REST

In any position you like, or need. If you do favour some resting positions over others: why is that?

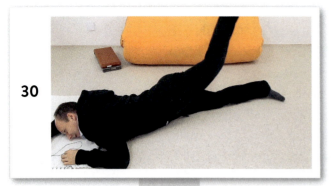

LIFT YOUR LEFT LEG TO ROLL OVER

Start with your head turned to the left, your left hand on top of your right hand. Actually, just place your hands somewhere close to your head, some place comfortable. Lift your left leg.

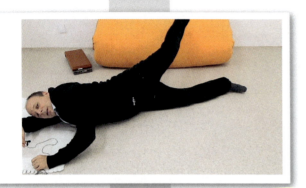

Lead with your left leg – on a pathway that will make it easy for you to gradually roll over onto your back. Put your right arm out of the way. Don't hurt yourself, don't sacrifice any part of yourself to achieve your goals. Help yourself feel comfortable.

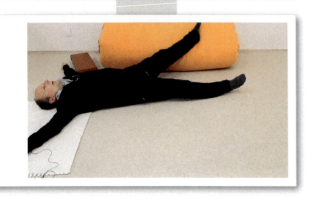

Then roll the same way back, as if you would play back a video in reverse, make the movement of rolling over reversible. Don't muscle your way back, be clever, use gravity, think of your skeletal system, your weight in different areas of your body (e. g. the weight of your leg, arm, head).

• •

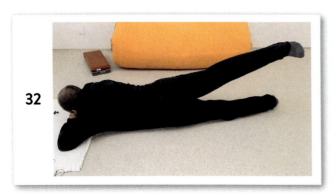

SAME ROLLING VARIATIONS ON THE OTHER SIDE

Try the same thing with your head turned to the right, leading with your right leg or right arm.

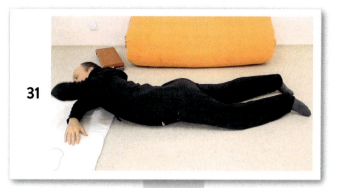

LIFT YOUR LEFT ARM TO ROLL OVER
Instead of leading with your leg, now lead with your left arm (or more precisely maybe: your left elbow).

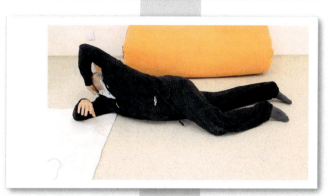

Explore. Find the easiest pathway. Feel, sense, move, think.

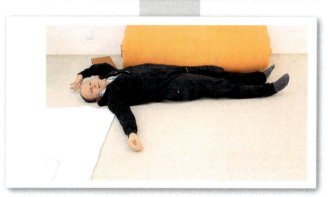

Once you successfully rolled over onto your back, think of how to get back onto your front side again. Try this many times, take every obstacle as an opportunity to improve. Continue until you feel satisfied with your movements. Don't strain. There's history to be re-written!

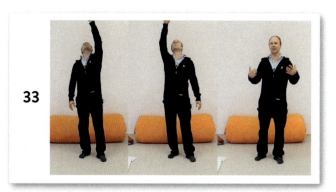

SIT AND STAND
Come to standing and see how it is.

Andy Heap — 7 months ago

Absolute genius

Alice Nird — 11 months ago

Fantastic class Alfons, thank you! My body feels so different that I can actually sit in the awkward position my computer is in to connect to my TV and write a comment. And thank you for the reminder sheet, that's a great help because I do need a prompt to remember the movements.

Fugi Cian — 3 months ago

Alfons is the best! <3

Penthesilea — 2 months ago

Excellent. Thank you

Rose-Marie Sorokin — 6 months ago

Wonderful!!!!

Tara Czutno — 6 months ago

Great to do in the morning. Thanks for all your videos. You are helping me save my life from fibromyalgia.

Bernadette Kozlowski — 8 months ago

Alfons, Have ben doing your videos each night... first I am sleeping better, second I went for a walk at the park last week and without trying to do anything different, noticed how much better my posture was and how much more self-aware I was. Enjoying being aware of the internal sensations of my body. Third, I am grateful to you for the moving meditation each evening!

Teresa Vega — 11 months ago

Hello from Spain. Thank you for your vídeos. Every time I do the exercises my eyesight improves so much.

Maria Mitea — 11 months ago

Ingeniouse :)

Phil Gardner — 11 months ago

Thanks Alfons - really liked how you wrapped everything together from the previous lessons. At a break in the middle, the shoulders felt very relaxed (as much as from the Freedom for stiff shoulder's lesson with Jeanette), and the flexion and extension on one arm and one elbow felt great - working with different muscles, vertebrae, etc. Nice lesson.

Maud v. — 11 months ago

Genial loosens area between shoulderblades,- great after bankart shoulder operation. Winning mobility back mami!

Leon Byng — 11 months ago

Thanks to you and your videos, I'm finally able to fold my body up from a standing position to a sitting floor position and get up from the floor by rotating hips and un-folding my body to stand.

I had a stroke 4 years ago and bit by bit I'm regaining flexibility and movement. I now explore my body position and knowing how the body is structured I can instantly well almost choose the best way to move. Thank You

rossana — 9 months ago

Thank you very much for this videos, beside the other benefits i get my vision more brite, i'm working with Bates metod and toghether with Feldenkrais it's accelereting the results!

Penthesilea — 2 months ago

Thanks for everything. You are simply the best.

All testimonial citations in this chapter are from publicly visible comments in the public comment section of my YouTube videos „TRY THIS SUN SALUTATION OF AWARENESS (MBSR, MINDFULNESS)", https://goo.gl/WJ9WqD and „YOUR WELLBEING AND SOMATIC EDUCATION", https://goo.gl/twR6sx, (December 9, 2017). I try to attribute as correctly as feasible, according to the official APA guidelines.

LESSON 9

Flexion & Extension In 16 Different Positions

*Life is a journey to be experienced,
not a problem to be solved.*

WINNIE THE POOH

PLEASE WORK THROUGH THE
VIDEO FIRST
TO BENEFIT FULLY FROM THIS
Workbook

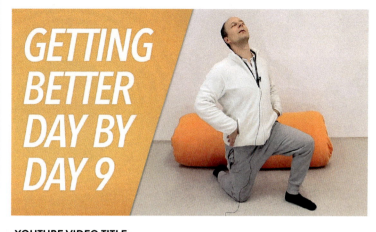

YOUTUBE VIDEO TITLE:
TRY THIS SUN SALUTATION OF AWARENESS (MBSR, MINDFULNESS)

Throughout the entire lesson (and the various starting positions) we will explore the following two movements: lowering the head and lifting the head (which will be flexion and extension regarding the spine). We have looked at these two movements extensively in the last eight lessons. Now we will transfer what we have learned so far into positions other than lying prone or supine. In every position this will feel different, and actually it will be quite different – even though the movements themselves are quite similar. New positions create new possibilities.

Take breaks as you need them. Always take breaks as an opportunity to check how you feel, what you sense, how you perceive the floor, the environment, what's different to before, to ask more questions.

TRANSFER

We use a variety of different positions to explore how to transfer movements from one position to another. Ultimately this is a learning process (or a reminder) of how to transfer the movements, the findings, the revelations and the benefits and so on, into our everyday lives, and how to benefit from the teachings in this course for a long time.

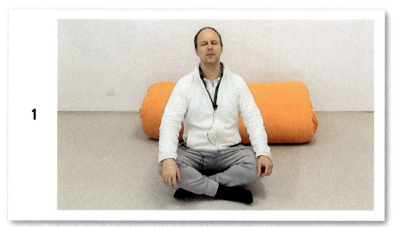

1

SIT CROSS-LEGGED

If you can't sit on the floor indian fashion without rounding your back, then help yourself with a hard cushion or something similar to sit on. Move through flexion and extension, as studied in great detail in the previous lessons.

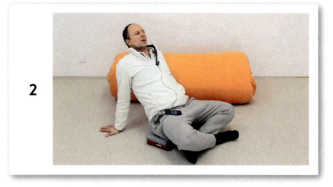

SIT CROSS-LEGGED, LEAN ONTO YOUR HANDS

If your wrists don't play along (=hurt) you can try leaning onto your fists. Again explore the same two movements, which in this position could be described as: sinking your head forwards and letting it slowly drop backwards. Always move your whole self (including your pelvis) not just your head. Think of what you've learned in the previous 8 lessons. With each new position explore and notice how these two movements are different than in the other positions.

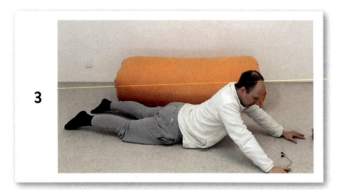

IN PRONE POSITION, LEAN ONTO YOUR HANDS

Put your hands wherever it makes sense to you. Prop yourself up with your arms extended. Continue with the exploration of the two movements.

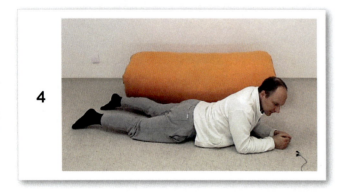

IN PRONE POSITION, LEAN ONTO YOUR ELBOWS

Make sure that your shoulders are free to let your spine move independently from your shoulders. Your shoulders should not restrict or define the movements of your spine. For a warm up you could try shoulder circles to free up your shoulder blades. Again, as in all positions in this lesson, explore the two movements of extension and flexion. Identify the peculiarities, restrictions, but also opportunities of this position. Are there details you can notice in this position but not in others? How is being propped up onto your elbows different from being propped up onto your hands with straight arms?

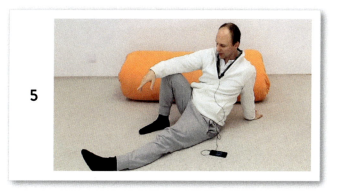

5

SIT WITH YOUR LEFT LEG EXTENDED, YOUR RIGHT FOOT STANDING, YOUR RIGHT ARM ON RIGHT KNEE, LEAN ON YOUR LEFT HAND

Be sure to actually lean on your left hand. This is the first asymmetrical position in this lesson. Find and follow the curved pathways that emerge from this. Note: if you look carefully enough you will be able to feel and find asymmetries in all previous positions.

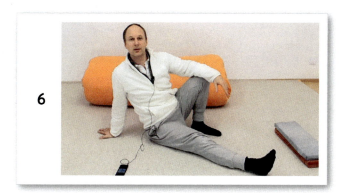

6

SIT WITH YOUR RIGHT LEG EXTENDED, YOUR LEFT FOOT STANDING, YOUR LEFT ARM ON LEFT KNEE, LEAN ON YOUR RIGHT HAND

Basically the same as before, but „on the other side". Compare with the curved pathways from the previous position. On this side the two movements might not only be flip-sided, but something completely else.

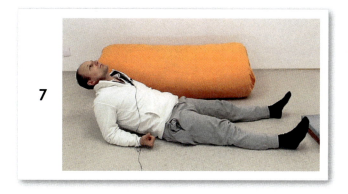

7

LYING SUPINE, LEAN ON ELBOWS

This is the opposite extreme of lying in prone position, propped up onto your elbows, as in [4]. In lying supine your head was pulled forwards by gravity, now in lying prone it's pulled backwards. Big difference. Try the two movements. Ask more questions.

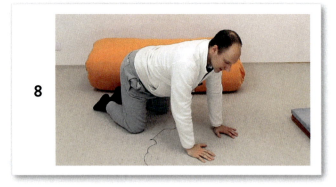

8

ON ALL FOURS
Place your knees properly under your pelvis, and your hands properly under your shoulders (not to the left, not to the right, not far out downwards, forwards etc). In this position the spine has a lot of freedom and is not restricted by (for example) the floor. Explore the two movements and move through your whole spine. Move your spine in a sequence starting with your eyes – head – neck – upper back – lower back – pelvis, or the other way round, or all at the same time, evenly timed and spaced.

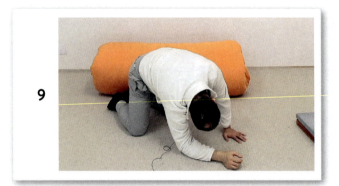

9

ON ALL FOURS, YOUR RIGHT ELBOW ON THE FLOOR
Again, this is a asymmetric position, find and follow the curved and almost spiralling/twisting pathways

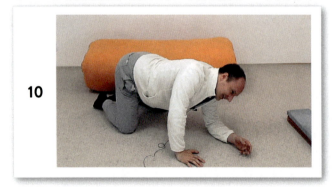

10

ON ALL FOURS, YOUR LEFT ELBOW ON THE FLOOR
Observe how and why this is different than before in step [9].

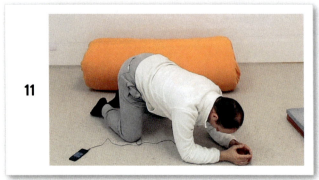

11

ON ALL FOURS, BOTH ELBOWS ON THE FLOOR
You can put your hands together or keep them elbow-width apart, just as you like. Explore. Feel how you perceive symmetry and centred movement now.

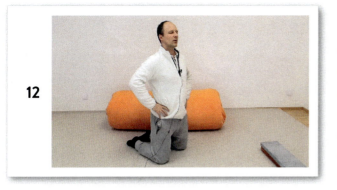

STAND ON KNEES, HANDS ON THE CREST OF THE ILIUM

While you bend forwards bring your elbows somewhat closer together in front of you. While you bend backwards bring your elbows somewhat closer together at your back. Do not bend over deeply, stick with flexion and extension. Keep your pelvis stable, don't overly sway your pelvis forwards and backwards.

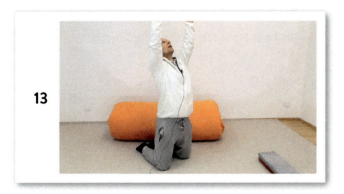

STAND ON KNEES, WITH HANDS UP

Keep your arms in place, fixed in space, while you lift and lower your head. Alternatively sway your arms a little bit forwards and backwards, follow them with your eyes and head. As always, let your whole spine (and pelvis) participate.

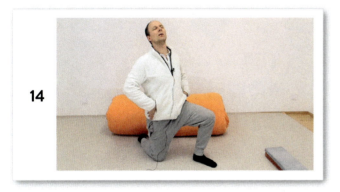

STAND ON RIGHT KNEE AND LEFT FOOT

Keep going with the flexion and extension movements. Try to feel on which side of your pelvis you are more stable, and on which side there is more possibility for movement. Look for a feeling of length throughout your whole spine. This is an asymmetrical position.

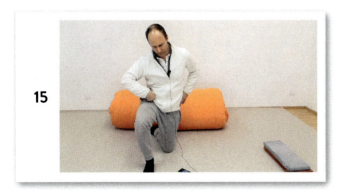

STAND ON LEFT KNEE AND RIGHT FOOT

Same as before, but with legs changed.

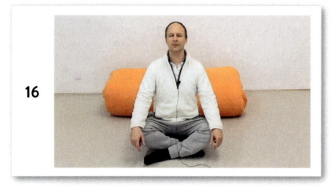

16

SIT CROSS-LEGGED
How is it compared to the beginning? Is sitting easier? Is the movement more clear, are some things more apparent? Can this be described as raised awareness?

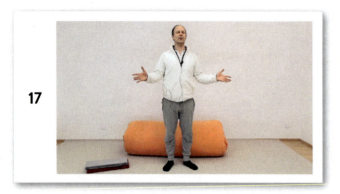

17

SEE HOW IT IS IN STANDING
Gently try the same thing in standing, then see how it is.

Philippe Berry 5 months ago
Thank you very much for all these videos! so real! so interesting! So natural! So funny!
Mille merci et respect!

Jean-marc Besenval 2 months ago
Hello Alfons I have just finished to do all your "getting better day by day" lessons. It has been a very nice trip and experience. I will watch and do more lessons. Unfortunately Austria is a bit far from where I live. Otherwise I could have come to take a lesson with you. Thank you very much for your work and passion. Keep on going !

Julie Fitzgerald 11 months ago
Thank you for creating your videos. Since discovering your channel, my personal movement practice and my teaching practice have benefited by what you are doing. It is exciting!

Liz Torres 10 months ago
Hi Alfons! Thank you so much for this introduction series, I have completed the exercises by practicing daily and I would like to share with you that I am feeling my body much better and realized how interesting it is to find different ways of movement and all the possibilities we have and also how much I have neglected my body.

During the first lessons and until around day 7 right after finishing the session I had a tingling sensation in the right leg, left arm, and neck... Funny :) but now After completing day 9 I don't have that sensation anymore. Anyway just want to thank you for sharing your knowledge with your great personality I wish I lived in your town to attend classes with you :P

Penthesilea 2 months ago
Thanks for everything. You are simply the best.

My dear reader, student, client, friend, follower, subscriber. Thank you so much for purchasing and using this workbook. Your support means the world to me.

I hope your study of this book does benefit (and will continue to benefit) yourself, your practice, and all the people your are connecting with.

As this is the last page in this book, may I bring your attention to my first book, „My Feldenkrais Book"?

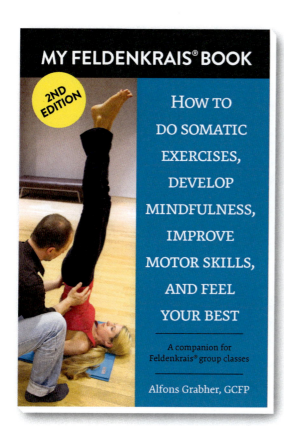

More info about this book, that book, and my other projects, and more on

WWW.MYFELDENKRAISBOOK.COM

„My Feldenkrais Book" is all about HOW to do Feldenkrais lessons (as opposed to WHAT to do). I try to convey the stance, the feeling, the bearing, of and when doing Feldenkrais lessons. Actually any type of somatic learning, experiencing or study, whatever the brand name. I think this book is brilliant, still a novelty of its own kind, and, if you don't have it already, I highly recommend purchasing it too.

All right. For me parting is always the most difficult thing to do. Especially from such a long, dear to me project like this workbook. We never know whether or not there will be a next adventure, a next big project, a next exciting thing to come into our lives.

But usually there is.

Cordially Yours,

Alfons

Vienna, December 2017

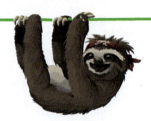

Made in the USA
Coppell, TX
01 December 2020

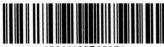
42644162R00071